Modern & Healthy

Body
Care

Recipes for Professional, Natural Skin and Hair Care Products

Karin Bombeli

First Edition

Modern and Healthy Body Care
Copyright © 1997 by the Somerset Company
All rights reserved

Although the author has exhaustively researched all sources to ensure the accuracy and completeness of the information contained in this book, no responsibility is assumed for errors, inaccuracies, omissions, or any other inconsistency herein. No liability is assumed with respect to the use or misuse of the cosmetic recipes and the occurrence of any unwanted skin or hair reactions.

Photographs by:
Thomas Bombeli, Bellevue, WA
Karin Bombeli, Bellevue, WA
Michael A. A. Keller, West Stock, Seattle, WA
Joe Polillio, Liaison International, New York, NY

Graphics by:
Thomas Bombeli, Bellevue, WA
Karin Bombeli, Bellevue, WA

Layout by:
Thomas Bombeli, Bellevue, WA

Edited by:
Peter Ansdell, Seattle, WA

Published by:
Somerset Company, P. O. Box 213, Bellevue, WA 98009
First Edition

ISBN 0-9658528-0-6
Library of Congress Catalog Card Number: 97-092195
Printed and bound in the United States of America

Acknowledgments

I wish to especially thank my husband, Thomas, for all his help, motivation and support. I also would like to express special gratitude to my editor, Peter Ansdell, whose editorial suggestions and corrections were very helpful. Additionally, I wish to acknowledge the following companies for their technical support and for generously providing samples to test new formulations: Brooks Industries, Inc. (South Plainfield, NJ); Henkel Corp. (Hoboken, NJ); Heterene, Inc. (Paterson, NJ); Protameen Chemicals, Inc. (Totowa, NJ); and TIC Gums (Belcamp, MD).

Dedication

This book is dedicated to all those who are looking for natural, healthy body care products, while still recognizing the achievements of modern cosmetic technology; to those who prefer individualized body care rather than cheap mass products, and to all those who just want the very best care for their skin and hair.

Contents

Preface

The Secret of Cosmetics

Introduction 10

Save Your Money as well as Your Skin and Hair

Equipment 13

Just Use Your Cooking Utensils

Methods 15

Fast, Easy, and a Lot of Fun!

Helpful Tips 17

Choose Your Basic Ingredient
Lemon Juice Against Alkalinity
No Cleansing Without Surfactants
How to Make an Emulsion
Essential Oils Are Really Essential
To Preserve or Not to Preserve?

Bath Oils 21

Bathing Adventures
Recipe 1: Invigorating Morning Bath
Recipe 2: Sensual Evening Bath
Recipe 3: Baths for Colds and Sores
Recipe 4: Baby Bath for Soft Baby Skin

Hand Cleansers 25

Hand Soaps for Every Day
Recipe 5: Soothing Hand Soap with Chamomile
Recipe 6: Fresh Citric Hand Soap for All Skin Types
Recipe 7: Hand Soap for Dry and Chapped Skin

Shower Gels 29

Shower Power
Recipe 8: Shower Gel with a Vigorous Effect
Recipe 9: Shower with the Scent of Roses
Recipe 10 and 11: Aromatherapy Shower Gels After a Busy Day
Recipe 12: Men's After-sport Shower Power
Recipe 13: Women's After-sport Shower Power
Recipe 14: Soothing Shower After a Day in the Sun

Face Cleansing Lotions and Toners 35

For Your Face Only
Recipe 15 and 16: Cleansing Lotion and Toner for Normal Skin
Recipe 17 and 18: Cleansing Lotion and Toner for Dry and
Sensitive Skin
Recipe 19 and 20: Cleansing Lotion and Toner for Oily Skin

After-sun Lotions 39

Tanning Needs Special Care
Recipe 21: Soothing After-sun Lotion with Herbs
Recipe 22: Nourishing After-sun Cream with Vitamins

Hair Shampoos 41

The Hair, Our Most Attractive Feature
Seven Tips for Healthy Hair and Scalp
Recipe 23: Herbal Shampoo for Normal Hair
Recipe 24: Lecithin Shampoo for Dry Hair
Recipe 25: Aromatherapy Shampoo for Oily Hair

Recipe 26: "Goodbye to Tears" Shampoo for Kids
Recipe 27: Shampoo and Conditioner All in One for Normal Hair

Anti-dandruff Shampoos 47

Natural Anti-dandruff Therapy
Recipe 28: Shampoo for Dry Dandruff
Recipe 29: Herbal Scalp Tonic for Dry Dandruff
Recipe 30: Shampoo for Oily Dandruff
Recipe 31: Herbal Scalp Tonic for Oily Dandruff

Hair Conditioners 51

Soft, Shiny, and Healthy Hair
Recipe 32: Herbal Conditioner for Normal to Dry Hair
Recipe 33: Vitamin Conditioner for Damaged Hair
Recipe 34: Herbal Rinse for Dry Hair

Ingredients 55

Basic Ingredients
Plant Distillates
Tinctures and Plant Extracts
Plant Oils
Vitamins
Other Botanical Ingredients
Surfactants
Emulsifiers
Essential Oils
Preservatives

Appendix 86

References
Supplier List
Addresses
Index
About the Author

Preface

Have you ever read the list of ingredients on the label of your shampoo or shower gel? – Doesn't it sound like the table of contents in a chemical textbook? – I remember a couple of years ago when I tried to understand what those chemical names really meant. I was quite frustrated. What was I actually using for washing my body and hair? – Were all those ingredients synthetic chemical products or were they just scientific names for natural products? Were all those ingredients necessary anyway? And, which of them were healthy and which were harmful? These questions made me decide to do some research and disclose some of the secrets of making cosmetics.

The Secret of Cosmetics

Surprisingly, these secrets were not as difficult to discover as the cosmetic industry would lead you to believe. I was able to quickly learn the basic formulas of cosmetics, and soon I was devising various ways of creating my own cosmetics. I also realized that creating my own cosmetics did not necessarily mean creating second class cosmetics. Instead, I was creating professional top quality products, which were exactly designed for my skin and hair.

Furthermore, my knowledge of the chemical and medical properties of cosmetic ingredients allowed me to unveil the technical terms on the labels and to sift the chaff from the wheat of these commercial products. And I can tell you, there is plenty of chaff on the market. Do not believe the promises in the advertisements, because many commercial cosmetics do not contain the valuable ingredients and do not deserve the term "natural product," which is often labeled on the bottle. Also, there are hundreds of cosmetics on the market containing substances, which have long been demonstrated in numerous clinical studies to be harmful for the skin.

Moreover, people with allergies often have trouble in finding a product without their specific allergenic agent, since most cosmetics contain a similar assortment of ingredients. However, by creating your own cosmetics, this will assure you that your product will be of a high quality with all the ingredients one often misses and without the ingredients one often dismisses.

Unfortunately, there are still many people who do not know that cosmetics can be self-made. Also, there are many people thinking that creating cosmetics can be difficult, costly, and time consuming, requiring the attendance of numerous classes. However, the opposite is true: creating cosmetics is easy, inexpensive, fast, and does not require any practical or theoretical courses.

This book shows you what natural shampoos, gels, lotions, face toners, and bath oils are made from, how easy it is to create them, how much money you can save, and how natural these products are. Without learning much theory, you will be able to create a top shampoo perfectly suited for your hair, a herbal shower gel with your preferred scent, or a creamy body lotion for any kind of skin type. This book also provides a rich source of information about the pros and cons of various chemical and natural ingredients.

For more than seven years, I have exclusively used my own cosmetics and I would never ever go back to a commercial product again. By adding some vitamins, along with pure aloe vera extract, and some lavender essential oil to your shampoo, you can feel certain that you will have a real natural product. Try it and have fun!

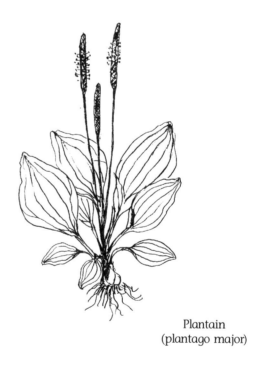

Plantain
(plantago major)

Introduction

For centuries, women and men have been interested in improving their appearance by constantly creating and using new cosmetics. At no time, however, has the use of cosmetics been so prevalent, nor has there been such a wide range of products to select from. This vast interest in skin and hair care is clearly demonstrated by the increasing marketing statistics and sales of cosmetic products.

Save Your Money as well as Your Skin and Hair

Whereas in 1980, only 4.6% of the total retail sales by broad merchandise lines in the USA were cosmetics, their contribution is now more than 15%. Similarly, the percentage of cosmetics in the total magazine and television advertising expenditures increased by more than 10%, which corresponds to a sum of more than $2 billion a year.

Thus, it seems evident that people pay more attention to their appearance by spending more money for more and better personal care products. Also, both women and men become more aware of the importance of more healthy and individualized skin and hair care. More and more people no longer want to use just any hair shampoo or skin care product, but instead want those that are customized to their type of hair and skin and which also improve the health of their hair and skin. Modern cosmetics are expected to not only contribute to your appearance, but also to your health. Furthermore, in the past few years, there has been a dramatic increase in the demand for natural products. Besides the general "back-to-nature" trend, many people realize that synthetic products do not always accomplish what they promise and often become responsible for newly found adverse reactions. Natural products, however, have been recognized to cause many less skin problems, and at the same time, actually improve the mildness of the product. Hence, the modern customer asks for healthy, natural, and individualized body care products of high quality, as well as obtaining those that are affordable.

However, although they think they know what to look for, most people do not know where to find it. Without knowing the properties and effects of each of the ingredients labeled on a cosmetic product, it is almost impossible to determine the quality of a product. Many of us will evaluate a product by its price and the promises in the advertisements. However, there are quality cosmetics and then there are others. While many products on the market are certainly mild and of good quality, there are a number of cosmetics, which do not contain any active ingredients, or they might have an inadequate concentration. Moreover, many products still contain ingredients known to be of high risk and may cause inflammations and other problems. This may be reflected by the remarkable number of more than 20,000 emergency room admissions a year in the USA due to cosmetic related side-effects.

This book, however, will not attempt to rate commercial cosmetics. It will tell you how to create your own body care products. They will be products that are modern, healthy, natural, and, of course, individualized. You will find 34 recipes to create your own liquid soap, shower gel, cleansing lotion, face toner, after-sun lotion, bath oil, shampoo, or conditioner.

So don't have any concerns, because creating your own cosmetics is easy. You do not need to be a chemist, nor to spend that much money and time. By contrast, after having obtained some ingredients, you will be able to produce many different body care products for yourself and your entire family in a very short time. Moreover, you will save a lot of money. A top-of-the-line hair shampoo of a prestigious brand can generally be priced up to $20.00. Nevertheless, many of these products do not contain the valuable ingredients, which one would expect for this price. On the other hand, a shampoo created by yourself, however, will only cost you between $3.00 and $5.00, including the bottle. At the same time, you can be sure that your shampoo does not contain any harsh cleansing agents, artificial colors, synthetic fragrances, worthless mineral oils, nor harmful preservatives, but only exclusively valuable ingredients, which have been prepared and selected by you. Your shampoo will receive only mild cleansing agents, precious oils, pure herbal tinctures, and natural essential oils, and will appear as a natural golden-brown color. Finally, you yourself will decide whether the shampoo will be preserved or not, and if yes, for how long and at which concentration.

Besides the principles of creating body care products, this book will tell you a lot about the effects and properties of natural and synthetic ingredients. This knowledge may not only inspire you to begin to try your own recipes, but also may convince you that your very own cosmetic products may be the products you will keep for a lifetime. They will be yours naturally.

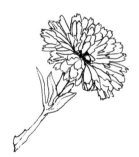

Marigold
(calendula officinalis)

Equipment

To mix your own shampoos, gels, lotions, and toners, you do not need many items, nor do you need to spend a lot of money. Assuming your kitchen is equipped with some basic cooking utensils, you will already be prepared to try your first recipes. First, you will need two glass jars holding about two cups (all recipes are calculated for a volume not larger than one cup).

Just Use Your Cooking Utensils

Plastic jars are not recommended, since their inner coating may soon get damaged upon frequent stirring. Such jars can no longer be disinfected properly and often become a source of bacterial contamination. Hence, glass is the preferred material. For measuring ingredients, a balance, scaled household spoons, and cups are ideal. Since essential oils and preservatives are added dropwise, a medicinal dropper is very useful. However, most essential oils are available in small glass bottles, which are already equipped with a dropper. Wooden spoons should not be used for stirring, since they are difficult to keep free from bacteria and often release small particles from their surface.

Thus, I recommend the use of a glass stick or a plastic spoon. To achieve complete homogenization and gelatinization of the mixture, an electric hand mixer (for small amounts) or a kitchen blender (for large amounts) is ideal.

Finally, a cosmetic container is needed for storing the products. Plastic is more useful than glass, since it can be squeezed and is unbreakable. Most packaging and bottle supply companies offer many different, practical containers. Of course, used cosmetic containers of commercial products or other bottles, which are not especially designed for cosmetics, are suitable as well.

Equipment

1. Two glass jars (two cup size)

2. Household measuring utensils

3. Medicinal dropper

4. Plastic spoon or glass stick

5. Electric hand mixer or kitchen blender

6. Plastic or glass cosmetic container

Methods

Mixing a shampoo, gel, lotion, or toner is easy. It should not take you more than 15 minutes, even as a beginner. First, clean and disinfect the glass jars, measuring utensils, and the cosmetic containers. Disinfecting is easily done by cleansing the containers with rubbing alcohol (contains isopropyl alcohol). It is available in drug stores. Discard the rubbing alcohol completely and rinse thoroughly with water.

Fast, Easy, and a Lot of Fun!

Then pour all the basic ingredients into the jar. These form the liquid base of a recipe and may include distilled water, teas, or decoctions. In most recipes, xanthan gum is added. Xanthan gum is a powder and acts as a natural thickener. It will readily dissolve, when sprinkled slowly into the water and stirred thoroughly with the hand mixer for about half a minute. If there are still some residual small flakes left, the mixture may then be warmed for a short time. The flakes should disappear. After a few minutes at room temperature, the mixture will become gelatinized and more viscous.

Lotions, such as after-sun lotions, face cleansing lotions, and conditioners, are based on an emulsion. Also, preparing an emulsion is easy and can be done within a few minutes. You will find a detailed description for preparing emulsions on page 18.

The next step is to add all the botanical ingredients one by one, and mix them again all together thoroughly with the electric hand mixer for about 10 to 20 seconds. As it is indicated in each recipe, botanical ingredients may include plant oils, herbal tinctures, proteins, vitamins, and lemon juice. Thereafter, all remaining ingredients, including the surfactants (cleansing agents), emulsifiers, essential oils, and preservatives are added. Stir the mixture gently with the glass stick or the plastic spoon. Mixing with the electric hand mixer is not recommended, since it may form too much foam. Voilà, your own cosmetic product is completed! It can now be poured into a nice cosmetic container or another suitable plastic bottle.

Method

1. Clean and disinfect all utensils with rubbing alcohol

2. Pour the distilled water into a jar. Sprinkle xanthan gum into the liquid while mixing continuously with the hand mixer

3. Add all botanical ingredients and mix again thoroughly with the electric hand mixer

4. Add all remaining ingredients and stir gently while avoiding the formation of foam

5. Pour the mixture into a cosmetic container

Helpful Tips

Choose Your Basic Ingredient

Usually, the basic ingredient of cosmetic products is distilled water. Distillation is necessary to remove sodium and other minerals, which can alter the beneficial effects of natural substances such as proteins, sugars, and fats. However, to achieve a more intense herbal basis in cosmetic products, distilled water can be replaced by tea. Basically, all teas are applicable for cosmetics! Just boil your favorite tea and use it as basic ingredient for your shampoo, shower gel, or lotion. Further information about the effects and properties of a special herb are listed in the chapter "Ingredients" (page 55). However, do not use tap water, but instead use distilled water for preparing the tea.

Lemon Juice against Alkalinity

The regular use of alkaline cosmetic products is well known as causing damage to the hydrolipid and acid mantle of the skin. This often induces skin irritations or inflammations that can predispose one to allergic reactions. Thus, it is important to maintain a mild acidity in all products. Although most recipes will already be neutral or slightly acid, the addition of lemon juice will assure a mild and natural acidity.

No Cleansing without Surfactants

Surfactants are cleansing agents, which are utilized in all personal care products that are used for cleansing and washing. The composition, properties, and effects of surfactants are explained in detail on page 71. In all recipes, the amount of surfactants necessary to achieve an optimal wash activity has been carefully calculated. Thus, if you want to prepare a larger amount, you need to increase the volumes of all ingredients proportionally. The ratio between the volume of the surfactants and the volume of all watery ingredients should not be changed. It should always be kept as indicated. A lower or higher amount of water will alter the concentration of the surfactants and consequently the optimal wash activity. For instance, if you want to omit one tablespoon of herbal tincture, you will have to replace it with one tablespoon of water. Similarly, if you want to use a smaller amount of surfactants, it will be necessary to reduce the amount of water by the same volume.

How to Make an Emulsion

An emulsion is a stable liquid mixture of oil and water. Normally, oil and water do not mix, but are kept separated. In the presence of an emulsifier, however, they form a creamy, homogeneous solution. In this book, an emulsion is used as a basis for face cleansing lotions, after-sun lotions and hair conditioners. Pour the oil or any other fatty ingredients, such as sheabutter, into a heat resistant glass jar. Then, add the emulsifiers (sorbitan stearate and polysorbate 60) and prewarmed (ca. 160°F, 70°C) distilled water, while mixing thoroughly with the mixer (only low speed) until the mixture becomes creamy. This may take up to five minutes. Let the mixture cool down (ca. 95°F, 35°C) and add all the remaining ingredients.

In certain recipes, a liquid emulsifier (polysorbate 80) can be added to stabilize essential oils and to allow fat soluble vitamins to dissolve better. Also, emulsifiers can be used to make bath oils dispersible in the water for bathing.

Essential Oils are Really Essential

Generally, the addition of essential oils can be varied individually. For instance, if a recipe contains ten drops of lavender and six drops of lemon essential oil, but you do not prefer lemon, then you certainly have the option to reduce the amount of lemon. Also, you can completely omit it and replace it by another essential oil.

However, the combination and total amount of essential oils should not largely differ from that indicated in the recipes. Both the blend and dosage of all essential oils have been carefully selected to achieve an optimal synergistic effect as well as to create a pleasant scent. When blended inadequately, essential oils can neutralize their beneficial effects on the skin and could smell strange and unpleasant. In addition, essential oils are not inexpensive and thus should be used sparingly.

To Preserve or not to Preserve?

Unpreserved cosmetic products can spoil due to the content of organic materials, which may allow the growth of different microorganisms. Spoiling means that natural substances such as proteins, sugars, and fats have become degraded, primarily by bacteria. Moreover, spoiled cosmetic products could be a source of skin infections. Thus, proper preservation is important.

However, preservatives can have unwanted effects when used at high concentrations or if one was trying to obtain a shelf life of two to three years as in commercial cosmetics. When used at such concentrations, many preservatives have been known to induce skin irritations and contact dermatitis. Making your own cosmetics, however, allows you to exclude preservatives or to choose mild preservatives at low concentrations, such as methyl- and propylparaben and diazolidinyl urea (DiU).

In a properly disinfected container, an unpreserved shampoo, gel, or toner containing essential oils, will not spoil until after about two months. Most essential oils have potent antibacterial, antiviral, and antifungal properties. Hence, the addition of a preservative to a shampoo, gel, or toner is only required, if a shelf life of more than two months is desired, or if the product contains lecithin or proteins, which may serve as "food" for bacteria. However, independent of their composition, lotions and creams should always be preserved, because they are usually stored in an open container and can thus be contaminated by one's fingers. If you do not want to use preservatives at all, then you should fill a lotion or cream in a dispenser, store it in the refrigerator, and try to use it up within two weeks. If formulations need to be preserved, 0.3% of a liquid preservative (Germaben-II) should be added. This concentration is the lowest concentration, which is still effective against microorganisms. Germaben-II contains parabens and DiU.

Helpful Tips

1. Use your favorite tea as a basic ingredient

2. Add lemon juice for natural acidity

3. Make sure that the surfactants are not diluted or concentrated

4. Take your time stirring an emulsion and do not use water that is too hot

5. Try your favorite essential oils, but use them economically

6. Use preservatives in lotions, creams, and products that contain lecithin and/or proteins

Bath Oils

One does not only bathe to wash oneself. Taking a bath can be more. It is a culture, a ceremony, or even a therapy. One bathes to relax, regenerate, care for one's skin, cure diseases and treat pains, or just to enjoy oneself. The benefits of oily ingredients in bath water has been recognized for hundreds of years. Chinese, Egyptian, and Roman civilizations have all had extensive knowledge of purifying and mixing herbal oils. Their use in medicinal and cosmetic skin preparations was very popular.

Bathing Adventures

Unfortunately, many commercial bath oils no longer contain plant oils but instead use cheap mineral oils as a basic ingredient. Mineral oils cannot be used in place of plant oils, since they are not able to penetrate the skin, but instead only stay on the skin surface. Hence, they have only a lubricant effect. Plant oils, however, readily penetrate the skin and are thus very nourishing and are gently refatting. In addition, plant oils have a good soothing effect.

Therefore, I strongly recommend using plant oils, no matter which one. Jojoba oil may be the best, since it will keep fresh longer than the other plant oils. When used within two months, preserving is not necessary, since the recipes contain vitamin E and different essential oils, both of which have good antibacterial activity.

Bath oils are either floating or dispersible. Floating oils do not contain an emulsifying agent and thus will not mix very well with water. They float on the surface of bath water and adhere to the skin only after one emerges from the bath. In the presence of an emulsifier, the oil becomes dispersible and combines with the water. Dispersible oils adhere to the skin when the bather is in the water. The following recipes provide dispersible oils. One half cup of these recipes is enough for about four to six baths.

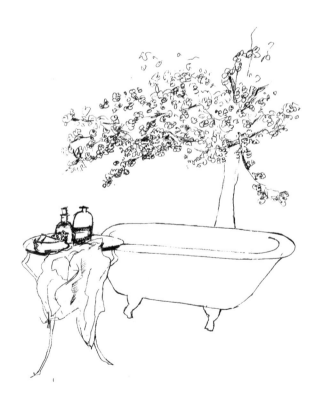

Invigorating Morning Bath

When did you last start the day with a bath, instead of a shower? This bath oil will make you feel fresh, fit, and ready for a long day. The combination of two precious plant oils including honey will leave your skin very smooth, soft, hydrated, and gently refatted. The ingredients for one half cup (120 ml) are:

Botanical Ingredients
1/4 cup (60 ml) Jojoba Oil
1/4 cup (60 ml) Almond Oil
1 tsp. (5 ml) Honey
1/4 tsp. (1.3 ml) Vitamin E
Emulsifier
1/2 tsp. (2.5 ml) Polysorbate 80
Essential Oils
35 drops Rosemary
30 drops Lemon
10 drops Sandalwood
10 drops Ylang Ylang

Sensual Evening Bath

This oil is the perfect ingredient for a relaxing and regenerating bath after a busy day. It contains a similar mixture of two valuable plant oils and honey, as described in the previous recipe. The bouquet is herbaceous, warm, deep, and more relaxing than refreshing. The ingredients for one half cup (120 ml) are:

Botanical Ingredients
1/4 cup (60 ml) Jojoba Oil
1/4 cup (60 ml) Soybean Oil
1 tsp. (5 ml) Honey
1/4 tsp. (1.3 ml) Vitamin E
Emulsifier
1/2 tsp. (2.5 ml) Polysorbate 80
Essential Oils
35 drops Lavender
25 drops Clary Sage
20 drops Neroli
10 drops Rose

Bath For Colds and Sores

This is an old folk remedy to cure colds and sores by steam baths, which are supplemented with herbal essences. All essential oils in this recipe are widely used in different balms and are known for their potent antiinflammatory properties. Their intense scent will help to relieve headaches, coughs, colds, and nasal congestion. A hot bath using this oil can also be very helpful for sore muscles and joints after sports and workouts. However, those who like the strong scent of juniper and peppermint do not need to wait until the next cold! The ingredients for one half cup (120 ml) are:

Botanical Ingredients
1/4 cup (60 ml) Jojoba Oil
1/4 cup (60 ml) Wheat Germ Oil
1 tsp. (5 ml) Honey
1/4 tsp. (1.3 ml) Vitamin E
Emulsifier
1/2 tsp. (2.5 ml) Polysorbate 80
Essential Oils
30 drops Peppermint
25 drops Juniper
25 drops Marjoram

Baby Bath for Soft Baby Skin

Since baby skin is usually very sensitive, skin care products need to be very mild. To achieve sufficent mildness, this formula contains a precious plant oil, which is combined with an essential amount of lecithin. Two mild surfactants are added to obtain a gentle cleansing effect. Provitamin B5 and calendula oil provide a good moisturizing and healing effect. I do not recommend using essential oils, because their intense scent may be too strong for babies. It has been shown that essential oils can induce headaches or can be harmful when swallowed. The ingredients for one half cup (120 ml) are:

Basic Ingredient
1/4 cup (60 ml) Chamomile Infusion
1/4 tsp. (1.3 ml) Xanthan Gum
Botanical Ingredients
1 Tbsp. (15 ml) Aloe Vera
1 Tbsp. (15 ml) Calendula Oil
2 tsp. (10 ml) Lecithin
1 tsp. (5 ml) Provitamin B5
Surfactant
2 tsp. (10 ml) Coco Betaine
1 tsp. (5 ml) Coco Collagen
Preservative
10 drops Paraben/DiU

Hand Cleansers

For quite a few years now, liquid hand soaps have largely replaced common bar soaps. This is not surprising, since liquid soaps are much more convenient and hygienic. They are easily dispensable and can additionally serve as refatting cream. Another benefit of liquid soaps is their mildness. Whereas bar soaps usually consist of harsh, aggressive, sodium-rich cleansing agents, liquid hand soaps contain modern semi-synthetic surfactants. These are generally less irritating due to their acidity and their low content of sodium.

Hand Soaps for Every Day

It has long been known that regular use of alkaline and sodium-rich products can result in damage to the hydrolipid and acid mantle of the skin. Although this acid mantle is usually restored after several hours or a day, it is thought that its repeated damage may induce skin irritations or make the skin more susceptible to allergies and solar radiation. Hence, all recipes in this book have an acid pH-value and are either sodium-free or contain only negligible amounts of sodium.

Unfortunately, there are some surfactants on the cosmetic market, which have also been found to cause skin problems. Some of them will be listed in the last chapter (page 71). For my recipes, I exclusively use surfactants which are derived from natural sources. Such products are known to be very mild. I have created three recipes for liquid hand soaps. Two of them are suitable for all skin types, while the other one is especially designed for dry and sensitive skin. All three recipes can be used to create herbal-based liquid soaps, which clean effectively and gently refat the skin. Before refilling the dispenser with new soap, make sure that the dispenser is washed and disinfected properly.

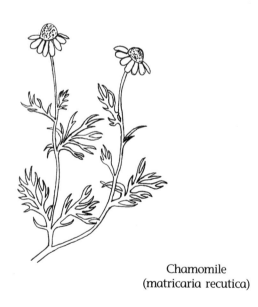

Chamomile
(matricaria recutica)

Soothing Hand Soap with Chamomile

This is a simple recipe for a basic hand soap. It contains mild surfactants, which have good cleansing capability. Because lecithin has a good refatting effect, your hands won't dry out even after using this soap many times a day. The ingredients for one cup (240 ml) are:

Basic Ingredients
1/2 cup (120 ml) Chamomile Infusion
1/2 tsp. (2.5 ml) Xanthan Gum
Botanical Ingredients
1 tsp. (5 ml) Lecithin
1/2 tsp. (2.5 ml) Lemon Juice
Surfactants
3 Tbsp. (45 ml) Coco Betaine
2 Tbsp. (30 ml) Polyglucose
Essential Oils
12 drops German or Roman Chamomile
Preservative
20 drops Paraben/DiU

Fresh Citric Hand Soap for All Skin Types

This hand soap is suitable for all skin types. It cleans very deeply and gently. Lecithin, aloe vera and witch hazel provide a pleasant refatting, moisturizing and soothing effect. Rosemary and citric essential oils give a fresh, citric, spicy aroma. The ingredients for one cup (240 ml) are:

Basic Ingredients
1/3 cup (80 ml) Distilled Water
1/2 tsp. (2.5 ml) Xanthan Gum
Botanical Ingredients
2 Tbsp. (30 ml) Witch Hazel Water
1 Tbsp. (15 ml) Aloe Vera
1 tsp. (5 ml) Lecithin
1/2 tsp. (2.5 ml) Provitamin B5
1/2 tsp. (2.5 ml) Lemon Juice
Surfactants
3 Tbsp. (45 ml) Coco Betaine
2 Tbsp. (30 ml) Polyglucose
Essential Oils
10 drops Grapefruit
8 drops Lemon
8 drops Rosemary
Preservative
20 drops Paraben/DiU

Hand Soap for Dry and Chapped Skin

This hand soap is particularly suitable for dry, parched, and chapped skin. It contains more lecithin and provitamin B5 than the previous recipe. After washing, the hands will be gently refatted and well moisturized. The ingredients for one cup (240 ml) are:

Basic Ingredients
1/3 cup (80 ml) Chamomile Infusion
1/2 tsp. (2.5 ml) Xanthan Gum

Botanical Ingredients
1 Tbsp. (15 ml) Witch Hazel Water
1 Tbsp. (15 ml) Aloe Vera
1 Tbsp. (15 ml) Comfrey Tincture
2 tsp. (10 ml) Lecithin
2 tsp. (10 ml) Wheat Germ Oil
1 tsp. (5 ml) Provitamin B5
1/2 tsp. (2.5 ml) Lemon Juice

Surfactants
1/4 cup (60 ml) Coco Collagen
3 Tbsp. (45 ml) Coco Betaine

Essential Oils
10 drops Lavender
10 drops Lemon
8 drops Vetiver

Preservative
20 drops Paraben/DiU

Shower Gels

Is there anything more stimulating than starting a new day by taking a shower accompanied by an aroma of roses or jasmine? And is there anything more relaxing than a shower with the delightful bouquet of natural herbs after a busy day or a workout in the gym? However, a shower gel should not only stimulate one's sense of smell, but also make one's skin feel fresh, clean, and moisturized.

Shower Power

Thus, a high-quality shower gel is more than a liquid and fragrant soap. It should contain mild cleansing and thickening agents, precious botanical extracts, and an important amount of essential oils. However, many if not most commercial shower gels lack herbal ingredients and often contain harsh and aggressive surfactants.

Hence, creating your own natural shower gel allows you to compose a very mild product of high quality. It will be very rich and have natural ingredients, which are harmonized to your skin type. It will also contain an exclusive blend of natural essential oils, rather than synthetic fragrances. After having used my own natural shower gels for many years now, my skin no longer feels tight and dry after a shower, but instead is smooth soft, and moisturized.

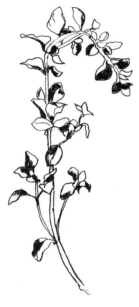

Marjoram
(origanum marjorana)

Shower Gel with a Vigorous Effect

This shower gel contains aloe vera as a herbal base for a good moisturizing effect. A selected blend of three different essential oils provides a fresh and spicy scent. Its stimulating effect makes one feel fresh and vigorous, which helps one to get started in the morning. It can be used for all skin types. The ingredients for one cup (240 ml) are:

Basic Ingredients
1/2 cup (120 ml) Distilled Water
1/2 tsp. (2.5 ml) Xanthan Gum
Botanical Ingredients
2 Tbsp. (30 ml) Aloe Vera
1 tsp. (5 ml) Lecithin
1/2 tsp. (2.5 ml) Honey
1/2 tsp. (2.5 ml) Lemon Juice
Surfactants
3 Tbsp. (45 ml) Polyglucose
3 Tbsp. (45 ml) Coco Betaine
Essential Oils
13 drops Juniper
8 drops Peppermint
6 drops Lemon
Preservative
20 drops Paraben/DiU

Shower with the Scent of Roses

This recipe gives a highly perfumed shower gel, which has a warm, floral, and romantic scent of roses. It is very mild and leaves the skin soft and smooth. Rose water has an excellent emollient, toning, and regenerating effect, which makes this shower gel especially suitable for sensitive and aging skin. The ingredients for one cup (240 ml) are:

Basic Ingredients
1/3 cup (80 ml) Distilled Water
1/2 tsp. (2.5 ml) Xanthan Gum
Botanical Ingredients
1/4 cup (60 ml) Rose Water
1 Tbsp. (15 ml) Aloe Vera
1 tsp. (5 ml) Lecithin
1/2 tsp. (2.5 ml) Honey
1/2 tsp. (2.5 ml) Lemon Juice
Surfactants
3 Tbsp. (45 ml) Polyglucose
3 Tbsp. (45 ml) Coco Betaine
Essential Oils
10 drops Rose or Rose Geranium
5 drops Sandalwood
Preservative
20 drops Paraben/DiU

Aromatherapy Shower Gels After a Busy Day

It is well-known that the intense scent of herbal oils can greatly influence mind and body. The following mixtures have a warm and soothing character. They can help you to relax after a busy day and make your skin clean, soft, and moisturized. One recipe should be considered for normal skin, while the other is especially designed for dry and sensitive skin. The ingredients for one cup (240 ml) are:

For Normal Skin

Basic Ingredients
1/2 cup (120 ml) Distilled Water
1/2 tsp. (2.5 ml) Xanthan Gum
Botanical Ingredients
1 Tbsp. (15 ml) Rose Water
2 tsp. (10 ml) Sage Tincture
1 tsp. (5 ml) Lecithin
1/2 tsp. (2.5 ml) Honey
1/2 tsp. (2.5 ml) Lemon Juice
Surfactants
3 Tbsp. (45 ml) Polyglucose
2 Tbsp. (30 ml) Coco Betaine
Essential Oils
10 drops Rose Geranium
8 drops Ylang Ylang
4 drops Clary Sage
4 drops Vetiver
Preservative
20 drops Paraben/DiU

For Dry and Sensitive Skin

Basic Ingredients
1/3 cup (80 ml) Distilled Water
1/2 tsp. (2.5 ml) Xanthan Gum
Botanical Ingredients
2 Tbsp. (30 ml) Orange Flower Water
1 Tbsp. (15 ml) Aloe Vera
2 tsp. (10 ml) Lecithin
1 tsp. (5 ml) Almond Oil
1/2 tsp. (2.5 ml) Honey
1/2 tsp. (2.5 ml) Lemon Juice
Surfactants
1/4 cup (60 ml) Coco Collagen
3 Tbsp. (45 ml) Coco Betaine
Essential Oils
9 drops Sweet Orange
8 drops Lavender
7 drops Palmarosa
6 drops Jasmine
Preservative
20 drops Paraben/DiU

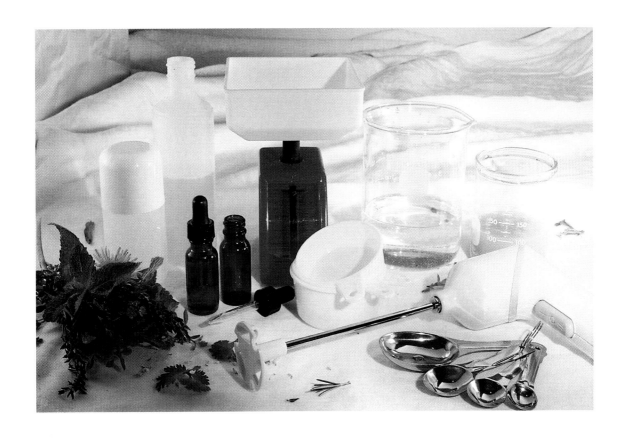

Discover unique recipes to create your own natural tonic waters,
herbal rinses, or scented bath oils

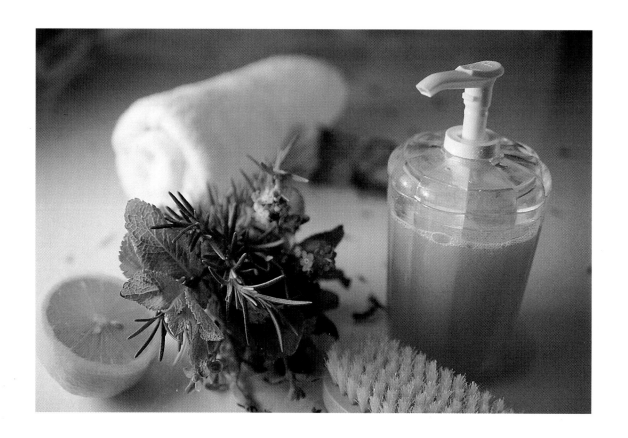

Naturally derived cleansing agents and different herbal extracts and essential oils make this liquid hand soap very mild with a fresh, citric aroma

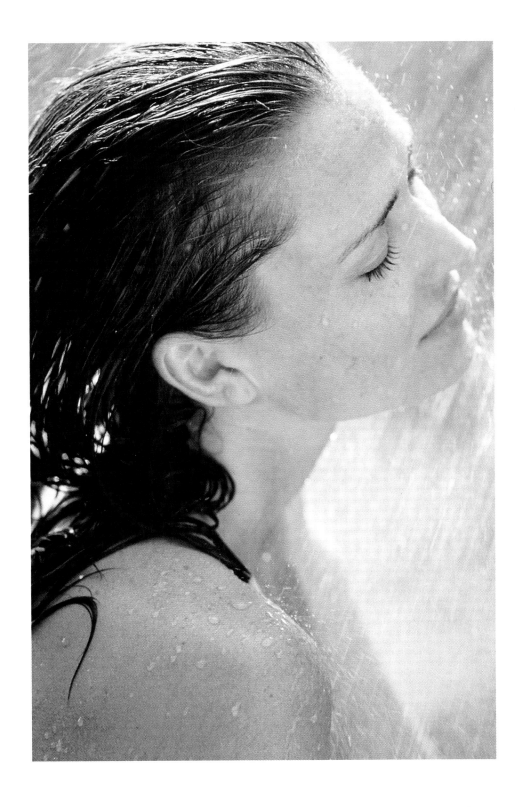

Self-made shower gels contain many valuable ingredients to keep the skin soft, moisturized, and gently refatted

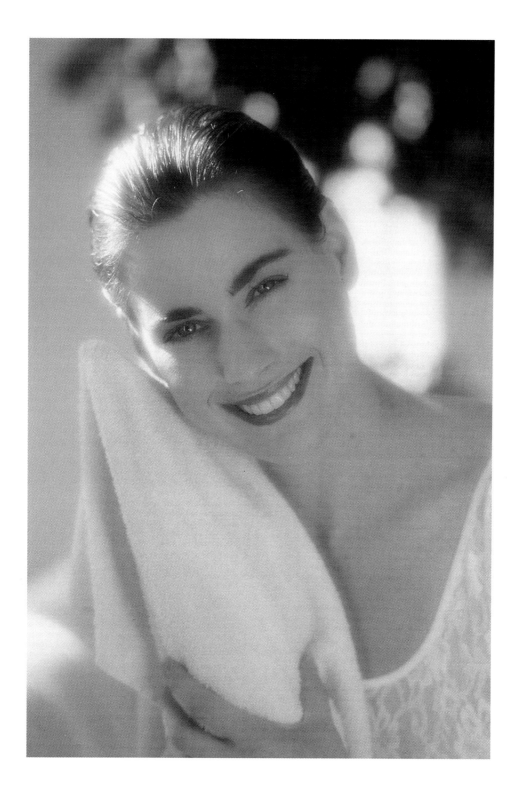

The regular use of herbal cleansing lotions and toners are
essential for a young and touchably beautiful skin

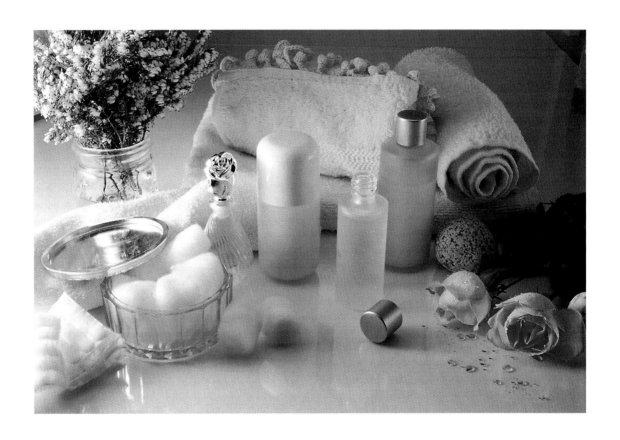

To optimize facial skin care, both cleansing lotions and toners
are especially designed for either normal, dry and sensitive, or oily skin

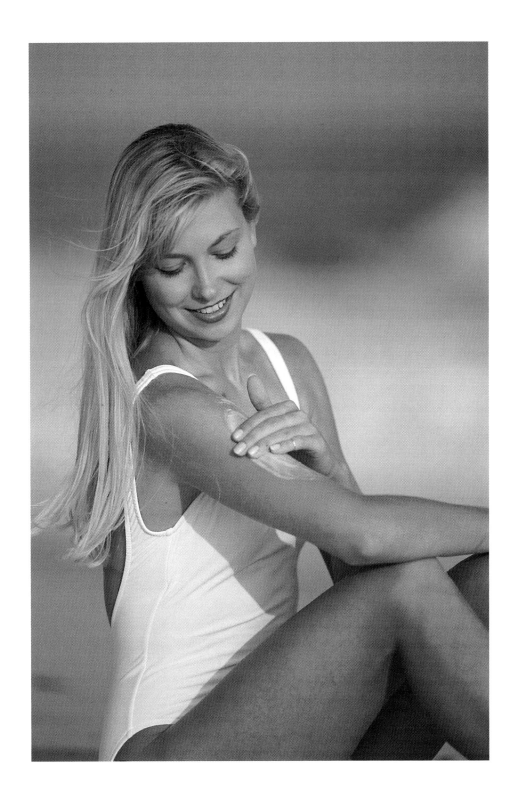

After sun bathing, the skin needs special care with a soothing,
regenerating, and deeply nourishing lotion or cream

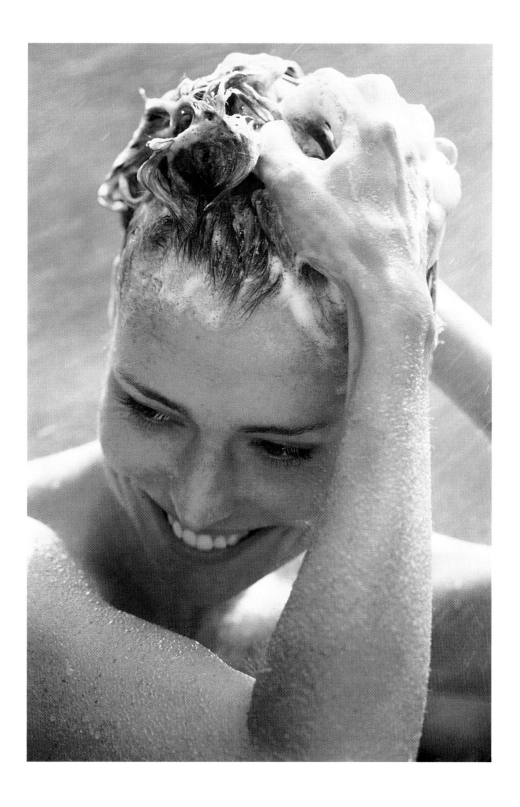

Natural hair shampoos cleanse very gently, nourish the hair and scalp,
and make the hair feel healthy and beautiful

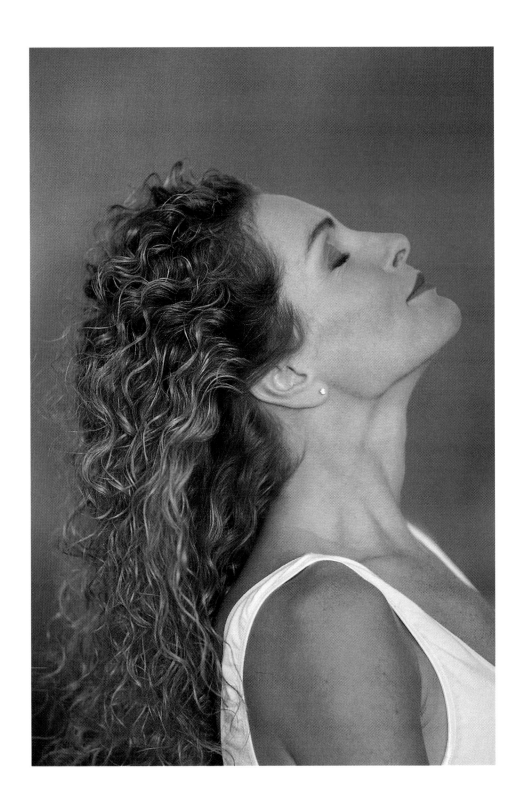

Dandruff can be treated successfully
with botanical ingredients

Men's After-sport Shower Power

This shower gel is especially designed for men. It contains a blend of very spicy, balsamic fragrances, which have quite a dry character. This makes it very refreshing and stimulating, as well as being ideal after sports and workouts. Due to its mildness and conditioning effect, it can be used for all skin types. It is also suitable as a hair shampoo. The ingredients for one cup (240 ml) are:

Basic Ingredients
1/3 cup. (80 ml) Distilled Water
1/2 tsp. (2.5 ml) Xanthan Gum
Botanical Ingredients
1 Tbsp. (15 ml) Sage Tincture
1 Tbsp. (15 ml) Aloe Vera
1 Tbsp. (15 ml) Stinging Nettle Tincture
1/2 tsp. (2.5 ml) Honey
1/2 tsp. (2.5 ml) Provitamin B5
1/2 tsp. (2.5 ml) Lemon Juice
Surfactants
1/4 cup (60 ml) Coco Collagen
3 Tbsp. (45 ml) Coco Betaine
1 tsp. (5 ml) Collagen Quat
Essential Oils
12 drops Rosemary
5 drops Marjoram
5 drops Ylang Ylang
4 drops Eucalyptus

Women's After-sport Shower Power

Similar to the men's recipe, this shower gel is very mild and can be used every day and for all skin types. Due to the addition of orange flower water, this gel has a refreshing and revitalizing effect, but the fragrance is warm and soft with a floral character. This shower gel leaves the skin soft, moisturized, and gently refatted. The ingredients for one cup (240 ml) are:

Basic Ingredients
1/3 cup (80 ml) Distilled Water
1/2 tsp. (2.5 ml) Xanthan Gum
Botanical Ingredients
2 Tbsp. (30 ml) Orange Flower Water
1 Tbsp. (15 ml) Aloe Vera
1 tsp. (5 ml) Lecithin
1/2 tsp. (2.5 ml) Avocado Oil
1/2 tsp. (2.5 ml) Honey
1/2 tsp. (2.5 ml) Lemon Juice
Surfactants
1/4 cup (60 ml) Coco Collagen
3 Tbsp. (45 ml) Coco Betaine
Essential Oils
12 drops Bergamot
8 drops Juniper
8 drops Jasmine
Preservative
20 drops Paraben/DiU

Soothing Shower After a Day in the Sun

Bathing in salt water or in the sun can rapidly dry out or irritate the skin. Thus, this recipe contains a special selection of soothing and antiinflammatory botanical ingredients. Lecithin and avocado oil are added to achieve a refatting and emollient effect. Salt residues in skin pores will be effectively removed by the combination of three mild surfactants. The ingredients for one cup (240 ml) are:

Basic Ingredients
1/2 cup (120 ml) Chamomile Infusion
1/2 tsp. (2.5 ml) Xanthan Gum
Botanical Ingredients
1 Tbsp. (15 ml) St. John's Wort Tincture
1 Tbsp. (15 ml) Witch Hazel Water
1 tsp. (5 ml) Lecithin
1 tsp. (5 ml) Avocado Oil
1/2 tsp. (2.5 ml) Provitamin B5
1/2 tsp. (2.5 ml) Lemon Juice
Surfactants
2 Tbsp. (30 ml) Coco Collagen
2 Tbsp. (30 ml) Coco Betaine
2 Tbsp. (30 ml) Polyglucose
Essential Oils
12 drops Lavender
8 drops Neroli
4 drops Vetiver
Preservative
20 drops Paraben/DiU

Face Cleansing Lotions & Toners

I n daily skin care, one pays most attention to one's face. It characterizes the human's individuality, expresses emotions, personality, character, age, and last but not least, beauty. Moreover, when exposed to wind, weather, dust, and dirt, face skin is unprotected all day long. In addition, it often has to tolerate make-up. Thus, it is undoubtedly the most strained and overburdened part of the entire human's skin.

For Your Face Only

Therefore, face products should not only cleanse effectively, but also be mild, moisturizing, and regenerating. However, common soaps can be aggressive, harsh, dehydrating, and are often inappropriate for sensitive skin types. Hence, I have created three different sets of face care solutions, which consist of a cleansing lotion and a corresponding toning water. They are designated for either normal, dry, or oily skin. Two of the lotions have an emulsion basis. Their preparation is described in detail on page 18. All toning waters contain different vitamins to achieve an optimal antioxidant and regenerating effect. Before using, the toner should be shaken to assure that the essential oils get mixed thoroughly. Before the toner is applied to the face, the skin should first be rinsed with cold or warm water to completely remove any residues of the cleansing lotion.

Cleansing Lotion and Toner
for Normal Skin

These formulas give both very mild and soothing solutions, which are ideal for daily use. The lotion cleanses very deeply and gently leaving the skin soft and smooth. In addition, it can be used as an effective make-up remover. The toner is a potent moisturizer, which makes the skin feel fresh and clean. Four vitamins provide a special nourishing and regenerating effect. The ingredients for one half cup (120 ml) are:

Cleansing Lotion

Emulsion Basis
1 Tbsp. (15 ml) Soybean Oil
2 tsp. (10 ml) Sheabutter
1 tsp. (5 ml) Sorbitan Stearate
1/2 tsp. (2.5 ml) Polysorbate 60
1/3 cup (80 ml) Hot Distilled Water
Botanical Ingredients
2 tsp. (10 ml) Calendula Tincture
2 tsp. (10 ml) Witch Hazel Water
1/2 tsp. (2.5 ml) Provitamin B5
1/4 tsp. (1.3 ml) Xanthan Gum
Surfactant
1 Tbsp. (15 ml) Polyglucose
Essential Oils
5 drops Lavender
4 drops Rose Geranium
Preservative
10 drops Paraben/DiU

Vitamin Toner

Basic Ingredient
3 Tbsp. (45 ml) Distilled Water
Botanical Ingredients
3 Tbsp. (45 ml) Orange Flower
Water
1 Tbsp. (15 ml) Ginseng Tincture
1 Tbsp. (15 ml) Aloe Vera
1/2 tsp. (2.5 ml) Provitamin B5
1/4 tsp. (1.3 ml) Vitamin C
1/4 tsp. (1.3 ml) Vitamin E
1/8 tsp. (0.7 ml) Vitamin A
Emulsifier
1/4 tsp. (1.3 ml) Polysorbate 80
Essential Oils
4 drops Lavender
3 drops Rose Geranium

Cleansing Lotion and Toner
for Dry and Sensitive Skin

Dry and sensitive skin can result from damage to the hydrolipid and acid mantle of the skin. The use of bar soaps or cheap cleansing gels with harsh surfactants should therefore be avoided. This recipe, however, is very mild. It contains a natural, mild surfactant, combined with a considerable amount of lecithin and plant oils. Rose water and aloe vera provide a good soothing effect. The ingredients for one half cup (120 ml) are.

Cleansing Lotion

Emulsion Basis
2 Tbsp. (30 ml) Avocado Oil
2 tsp. (10 ml) Sheabutter
1 tsp. (5 ml) Sorbitan Stearate
1/2 tsp. (2.5 ml) Polysorbate 60
1/4 tsp. (1.3 ml) Vitamin E
1/3 cup (80 ml) Hot Distilled Water
Botanical Ingredients
1 Tbsp. (15 ml) Rose Water
2 tsp. (10 ml) Aloe Vera
1/2 tsp. (2.5 ml) Provitamin B5
1/2 tsp. (2.5 ml) Lecithin
1/4 tsp. (1.3 ml) Xanthan Gum
Surfactant
1 Tbsp. (15 ml) Coco Collagen
Essential Oils
5 drops Lavender
3 drops Jasmine
Preservative
10 drops Paraben/DiU

Soothing Toner

Basic Ingredient
2 Tbsp. (30 ml) Distilled Water
Botanical Ingredients
3 Tbsp. (45 ml) Rose Water
1 Tbsp. (15 ml) Orange Flower Water
1 Tbsp. (15 ml) Aloe Vera
2 tsp. (10 ml) Chamomile Tincture
1 tsp. (5 ml) Avocado Oil
1/2 tsp. (2.5 ml) Provitamin B5
1/4 tsp. (1.3 ml) Vitamin E
1/8 tsp. (0.7 ml) Vitamin A
Emulsifier
1/4 tsp. (1.3 ml) Polysorbate 80
Essential Oils
4 drops Lavender
3 drops Jasmine

Cleansing Lotion and Toner
for Oily Skin

Oily skin is caused by highly active or inflamed sebaceous glands, and is often accompanied by acne. Hence, these recipes contain a relatively high amount of witch hazel water and burdock herbal tincture, which exert excellent antiinflammatory and soothing effects. Both the lotion and the toner contain only a minimal amount of fatty ingredients. The ingredients for one half cup (120 ml) are.

Cleansing Lotion

Basic Ingredients
1/4 cup (60 ml) Distilled Water
1/4 tsp. (1.3 ml) Xanthan Gum
Botanical Ingredients
2 Tbsp. (30 ml) Witch Hazel Water
2 tsp. (10 ml) Burdock Tincture
2 tsp. (10 ml) Jojoba Oil
1/2 tsp. (2.5 ml) Provitamin B5
Surfactant
2 Tbsp. (30 ml) Coco Betaine
Essential Oils
5 drops Lemon
3 drops Peppermint
Preservative
10 drops Paraben/DiU

Nourishing Toner

Basic Ingredient
1/4 cup. (60 ml) Chamomile
Infusion
Botanical Ingredients
2 Tbsp. (30 ml) Witch Hazel Water
1 Tbsp. (15 ml) Burdock Tincture
1 Tbsp. (15 ml) Sage Tincture
1/2 tsp. (2.5 ml) Provitamin B5
1/4 tsp. (1.3 ml) Vitamin E
1/4 tsp. (1.3 ml) Vitamin C
1/8 tsp. (0.7 ml) Vitamin A
Emulsifier
1/4 tsp. (1.3 ml) Polysorbate 80
Essential Oils
5 drops Lemon
3 drops Peppermint

After-sun Lotions

While over two generations ago, everything was done to assure that the skin was exposed to the sun as little as possible, today sunbathing is still very fashionable. Although modern sunscreens provide sufficient protection against sunburns, they do not reduce premature skin aging, dehydration of the skin, and the occurrence of sun-induced skin cancer. Extensive sun exposure can leave the skin dry, chapped, less elastic, and often slightly inflamed.

Tanning Needs Special Care

Therefore, after-sun skin care is as important as pre-sun skin care. This includes sufficient drinking of water and the application of a skin gel or lotion, which is mild, nourishing, moisturizing, and also refatting. In addition, it should exert soothing and antiinflammatory activities. To achieve all these properties, after-sun skin formulations need to be of high-quality, consisting of exclusive, precious ingredients.

To meet these high standards, I have created two luxurious after-sun lotions, which contain very valuable oils, well-selected botanical ingredients, and considerable amounts of proteins and vitamins. These should help to alleviate the adverse effects of solar radiation and maintain young and healthy skin. Like face cleansing lotions, after-sun lotions consist of an emulsion basis. Its preparation is described on page 18.

Soothing After-sun Lotion With Herbs

To obtain a good nourishing, healing, and moisturizing effect, this recipe contains apricot kernel oil and sheabutter. Aloe vera, witch hazel, vitamin E, and provitamin B5 provide potent antiinflammatory and antioxidant activities, respectively. Soy protein supports tissue regeneration and prevents dehydration. When applied to the skin, the lotion feels very soothing. It leaves the skin soft, moisturized, and gently refatted. The ingredients for one cup (240 ml) are:

Emulsion Basis
2 Tbsp. (30 ml) Apricot Kernel Oil
1 Tbsp. (15 ml) Sheabutter
1 Tbsp. (15 ml) Sorbitan Stearate
1 tsp. (5 ml) Vitamin E
1/4 tsp. (1.3 ml) Polysorbate 60
3/4 cup (180 ml) Hot Distilled Water
Botanical Ingredients
1 Tbsp. (15 ml) Aloe Vera
1 Tbsp. (15 ml) Witch Hazel Water
2 tsp. (10 ml) St. John's Wort Tincture
2 tsp. (10 ml) Soy Protein
1 tsp. (5 ml) Provitamin B5
1/4 tsp. (1.3 ml) Xanthan Gum
Essential Oils
10 drops Neroli
8 drops Lavender
Preservative
20 drops Paraben/DiU

Nourishing After-sun Cream With Vitamins

This recipe gives a cream. Due to its higher consistency, it is better dispensable and easier to apply to the face. Although it uses different herbal ingredients, this formulation has similar moisturizing and healing properties as the previous recipe. However, it has a more intense nourishing effect due to the addition of four vitamins. Since vitamin A is sensitive to light, this lotion should not be applied before, but exclusively after sun exposure. The ingredients for one half cup (120 ml) are:

Emulsion Basis
4 tsp. (20 ml) Wheat Germ Oil
1 Tbsp. (15 ml) Sheabutter
1 Tbsp. (15 ml) Sorbitan Stearate
1/2 tsp. (2.5 ml) Vitamin E
1/4 tsp. (1.3 ml) Polysorbate 60
1/3 cup (80 ml) Hot Distilled Water
Botanical Ingredients
1 Tbsp. (15 ml) Aloe Vera
2 tsp. (10 ml) Ginseng Tincture
1 tsp. (5 ml) Soy Protein
1/2 tsp. (2.5 ml) Provitamin B5
1/4 tsp. (1.3 ml) Vitamin C
1/8 tsp. (0.7 ml) Vitamin A
1/8 tsp. (0.7 ml) Xanthan Gum
Essential Oils
6 drops Lavender
5 drops German Chamomile
Preservative
10 drops Paraben/DiU

Hair Shampoos

Practically for all times, women and men have been concerned about their hair. Considered as the most important feature of the body, the hair has had many different ways tried to modify and beautify by brushing, grooming, coloring, cutting, waving, and bleaching. Moreover, the hair is an expressive secondary sexual characteristic and plays an important part in the psychological contacts of people in life. It influences one's complexion and personality and its condition may either attract and create a sympathetic reaction or may repel and create an adverse reaction. Many people thus pay a lot of attention to their hair care.

The Hair, Our Most Attractive Feature

The hair consists of three structures: the cuticle, cortex, and medulla. The cuticle is the outer layer, which is formed of overlapping scales. It is important for hair appearance, manageability, and shine. An undamaged cuticle has a smooth surface, which allows reflection of light, and gives the shine associated with healthy hair. Disruption of these scales is the first step in permanent hair coloring or waving. The consequences of disrupted cuticles are: rough surface, loss of shine, split ends, and static electricity.

The cortex forms the intermediate layer. It contains melanin, the natural hair dye, and is responsible for the hair's elasticity. The medulla is the innermost layer, which is very resistant and explains why there is a need for harsh chemicals to apply permanent dyeing or waving. Such deep defects may, however, never have a cure.

For a long time, shampoos were used solely for cleansing hair, but their range of functionality has extended considerably in recent years. A good shampoo is not only expected to cleanse, care, and condition the hair, but also be able to treat special hair and scalp problems. Whereas many commercial shampoos on the market can accomplish these postulations, numerous dermatological studies, however, have demonstrated that more than 5% of all commercial shampoos in the USA, produce clinically relevant side-effects; and it is very likely that the number of undetected cases may be much higher. Most substances that are found to be responsible, are synthetic fragrances, harsh surfactants, conditioning and coloring agents, and preservatives.

Thus, the significant increasing demand for natural cosmetic products over the last few years cannot be considered as a new fashion trend promoted by some companies to augment their sales. Rather, more and more people have become aware of the benefits of natural-based body and hair care products. Hair shampoos, containing natural ingredients such as herbal tinctures, vitamins, phospholipids, essential oils, and protein- or sugar-based surfactants will not do any harm to the hair, nor will they cause any irritations to the scalp. By contrast, they provide good care for the hair and are also capable of repairing damaged hair. However, to maintain healthy hair and scalp, additional factors should be considered as well, as described on the next page.

The following recipes will provide very mild, natural shampoos. Dependent on the quality of the hair and scalp, the herbal ingredients, oils, and surfactants will vary considerably. Now, let's create your own natural shampoo. Your hair will be thankful.

Seven Tips for Healthy Hair and Scalp

1. Use mild all-natural shampoos as shown in this book. "Synthetic" shampoos are often aggressive.

2. Use water not warmer than 104°F (40°C) for hair washing. The warmer the water, the more irritable becomes the skin.

3. Use hairbrushes with soft bristles and brush with soft strokes. Harsh brushing irritates the scalp and causes weathering.

4. Protect the hair from intensive solar radiation. Sun exposure dehydrates the hair causing hair breakage.

5. After swimming in salt water, rinse the hair thoroughly with fresh water. Salt residues will damage the hair cuticles.

6. Have second thoughts when considering to wave, bleach, or dye your hair. All these techniques damage the hair.

7. Do not blow dry your hair either too hot or too long. The hair will become desiccated and fragile.

Herbal Shampoo for Normal Hair

This shampoo is very mild and cleanses gently. It can be used every day. The generous addition of herbs, honey, and protein-based surfactants provides a very natural formula. It will deeply nourish both the hair and the scalp. Regular use will result in healthy, shiny, and beautiful looking hair. The essential oils are blended for a mild, herbaceous scent. You may add a personal touch by replacing distilled water with your favorite tea. The ingredients for one cup (240 ml) are:

Basic Ingredients
1/2 cup. (120 ml) Distilled Water
1/2 tsp. (2.5 ml) Xanthan Gum
Botanical Ingredients
1 Tbsp. (15 ml) Birch Tincture
1 Tbsp. (15 ml) Stinging Nettle Tincture
1/2 tsp. (2.5 ml) Provitamin B5
1/2 tsp. (2.5 ml) Honey
1/2 tsp. (2.5 ml) Lemon Juice
Surfactants
3 Tbsp. (45 ml) Polyglucose
3 Tbsp. (45 ml) Coco Betaine
1/2 tsp. (2.5 ml) Collagen Quat
Essential Oils
12 drops Lavender
10 drops Lemon
7 drops Palmarosa

Lecithin Shampoo for Dry Hair

Dry hair often results from shampoos with harsh surfactants, which remove the sebum completely, leaving the hair dry, rough, and with split ends. Therefore, this recipe contains a high amount of lecithin and rose water. They will effectively refat, moisturize, and reduce weathering. Although the shampoo is very mild, dry hair should not be washed too often. Hair should have time for refatting. Do not use hot blow drying. It will dry out the scalp. The ingredients for one cup (240 ml) are:

Basic Ingredients
1/4 cup (60 ml) Distilled Water
1/2 tsp. (2.5 ml) Xanthan Gum
Botanical Ingredients
2 Tbsp. (30 ml) Rose Water
1 Tbsp. (15 ml) Aloe Vera
1 Tbsp. (15 ml) Stinging Nettle Tincture
2 tsp. (10 ml) Lecithin
1/2 tsp. (2.5 ml) Provitamin B5
1/2 tsp. (2.5 ml) Lemon Juice
Surfactants
1/4 cup (60 ml) Coco Collagen
3 Tbsp. (45 ml) Coco Betaine
1 tsp. (5 ml) Collagen Quat
Essential Oils
8 drops Rose
6 drops Sandalwood
Preservative
20 drops Paraben/DiU

Aromatherapy Shampoo for Oily Hair

Greasy hair is caused by highly active or inflamed sebaceous glands (seborrhea). Hence, this shampoo does not contain any plant oils, but instead has three different herbal tinctures, which are very soothing and have good antiinflammatory activity. All three essential oils are known to reduce seborrhea. The effectiveness of this shampoo can be further improved when it is gently worked into lather and then is left to sit for a moment. The ingredients for one cup (240 ml) are:

Basic Ingredients
1/3 cup (80 ml) Distilled Water
1/2 tsp. (2.5 ml) Xanthan Gum
Botanical Ingredients
1 Tbsp. (15 ml) Sage Tincture
1 Tbsp. (15 ml) Birch Tincture
1 Tbsp. (15 ml) Stinging Nettle Tincture
1/2 tsp. (2.5 ml) Provitamin B5
1/2 tsp. (2.5 ml) Lemon Juice
Surfactants
3 Tbsp. (45 ml) Polyglucose
3 Tbsp. (45 ml) Coco Betaine
1/4 tsp. (1.3 ml) Collagen Quat
Essential Oils
12 drops Bergamot
8 drops Rose Geranium
7 drops Ylang Ylang

"Goodbye to Tears" Shampoo for Kids

Along with every other shampoo described in this book, this shampoo is not eye-irritating due to its natural surfactants. It is very mild and suits all hair types. Generally, in products for infants, essential oils should not be used at too high a concentration, since their intense scent may induce headaches or sickness. Thus, the concentration of essential oils is intentionally kept very low, which results in an almost neutral odor. The ingredients for one cup (240 ml) are:

Basic Ingredients
1/2 cup (120 ml) Distilled Water
1/2 tsp. (2.5 ml) Xanthan Gum
Botanical Ingredients
2 Tbsp. (30 ml) Aloe Vera
1/2 tsp. (2.5 ml) Lecithin
1/2 tsp. (2.5 ml) Lemon Juice
Surfactants
3 Tbsp. (45 ml) Coco Collagen
2 Tbsp. (30 ml) Coco Betaine
Essential oils
8 drops Sweet Orange
6 drops Lavender
Preservative
20 drops Paraben/DiU

Shampoo and Conditioner All in One for Normal Hair

The hair is conditioned best if it is treated with an exclusive conditioner. However, for normal, unproblematic hair, a sufficient conditioning effect may also be achieved using a shampoo, which contains conditioning agents. Such an effect can be obtained by a higher acidity, a small amount of plant oils, and a higher concentration of cationic surfactants. The ingredients for one cup (240 ml) are:

Basic Ingredients
1/2 cup (120 ml) Distilled Water
1/2 tsp. (2.5 ml) Xanthan Gum

Botanical Ingredients
1 Tbsp. (15 ml) Stinging Nettle Tincture
1 Tbsp. (15 ml) Burdock Tincture
1 Tbsp. (15 ml) Lemon Juice
1/2 tsp. (2.5 ml) Provitamin B5
1/2 tsp. (2.5 ml) Honey
1/2 tsp. (2.5 ml) Jojoba Oil

Surfactants
3 Tbsp. (45 ml) Polyglucose
3 Tbsp. (45 ml) Coco Betaine
1 tsp. (5 ml) Collagen Quat

Essential Oils
12 drops Peppermint
10 drops Rosemary

Anti-dandruff Shampoos

Dandruff is the result of excessive scaling of the horny layer of the skin of the scalp. However, the amount of scaling, which is usually regarded as bothersome, varies individually. Generally, dandruff is recognized when scales are visible and fall off. The cause of dandruff is not known. It usually begins to emerge at puberty and ends with old age. Interestingly, many people notice a significant decline in the summer months. Indeed, the horny cell production has been found to decrease during that time, but the reason for this seasonal variation is not evident.

Natural Anti-dandruff Therapy

Dandruff can be divided into an oily and a dry form. However, there are basically no different causes of dandruff. It just means that dandruff can occur either on a dry or an oily scalp. Thus, anti-dandruff shampoos should be formulated differently, either for a dry or an oily scalp. If the scalp, however, shows eczema-like indications, it is necessary to consult a dermatologist, since normal dandruff should never be associated with signs of inflammation.

Dandruff can be treated in two ways, either by removing the scales or by suppressing the excessive scale production of the horny cells. Scales are removed by shampooing. Unfortunately, within three to four days, the quantity of scales will return to the original level. Consequently, effective anti-dandruff therapy tries to additionally reduce scale production. In commercial products, this is achieved by different cytostatic drugs, such as selenium sulfide, zinc pyrithione, salicylic acid, or coal tar.

There are also, however, some natural substances which provide an effective anti-dandruff therapy. These include different herbal tinctures, such as burdock, sage, althea, birch, and stinging nettle, and also essential oils, such as lemon, rosemary, clary sage, ylang ylang, tea tree, and neroli. In addition, vitamin C and provitamin B5 have been found to be valuable ingredients in the treatment of dandruff.

For both dry and oily dandruff, I have created a shampoo as well as a tonic water for the scalp. Tonic waters are generally more effective than shampoos, since they are not rinsed out and remain longer on the scalp.

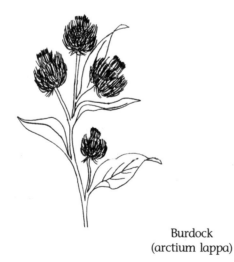

Burdock
(arctium lappa)

Shampoo for Dry Dandruff

This shampoo contains lecithin, jojoba oil, and three different herbal tinctures, which help to refat, moisturize and lubricate the hair. As a basic ingredient, I recommend a chamomile infusion instead of distilled water. This augments the moisturizing effect and soothes the irritated scalp. To improve the efficacy of the ingredients, massage the shampoo gently into the scalp and let it sit for a moment. The ingredients for one cup (240 ml) are.

Basic Ingredients
1/3 cup (80 ml) Chamomile Infusion
1/2 tsp. (2.5 ml) Xanthan Gum
Botanical Ingredients
1 Tbsp. (15 ml) Stinging Nettle Tincture
1 Tbsp. (15 ml) Birch Tincture
1 Tbsp. (15 ml) Aloe Vera
2 tsp. (10 ml) Lecithin
1 tsp. (5 ml) Jojoba Oil
1/2 tsp. (2.5 ml) Provitamin B5
1/4 tsp. (1.3 ml) Vitamin C
Surfactants
1/4 cup (60 ml) Coco Collagen
3 Tbsp. (45 ml) Coco Betaine
1 tsp. (5 ml) Collagen Quat
Essential Oils
14 drops Neroli
7 drops Rose
Preservative
20 drops Paraben/DiU

Herbal Scalp Tonic for Dry Dandruff

Tonic waters are very helpful additional solutions for intensifying anti-dandruff therapy. They are massaged into a dry or wet scalp and are not rinsed out. Hence, vitamins and herbal ingredients stay longer on the scalp for a more intense effect. The scalp will be effectively moisturized, and refatted. This recipe is based on a peppermint infusion, which helps to soothe the scalp and relieve itching. The ingredients for one half cup (120 ml) are.

Basic Ingredients
1/3 cup (80 ml) Peppermint Infusion
Botanical Ingredients
2 Tbsp. (30 ml) Aloe Vera
1 Tbsp. (15 ml) Stinging Nettle Tincture
1/2 tsp. (2.5 ml) Lecithin
1/2 tsp. (2.5 ml) Avocado Oil
1/4 tsp. (1.3 ml) Vitamin C
1/4 tsp. (1.3 ml) Vitamin E
1/4 tsp. (1.3 ml) Provitamin B5
1/8 tsp. (0.7 ml) Vitamin A
Emulsifier
1/4 tsp. (1.3 ml) Polysorbate 80
Essential Oils
4 drops Sage
3 drops Peppermint
Preservative
10 drops Paraben/DiU

Shampoo for Oily Dandruff

Oily dandruff needs more frequent treatment than dry dandruff. The excessive production of sebum often induces bacterial growth, which causes inflammations of the scalp. Therefore, this recipe contains different herbal tinctures, which are known for their good antibacterial and defatting effect. Tinctures also contain a small amount of alcohol, which is an excellent disinfecting and defatting agent. The shampoo is very mild and can be used daily. The ingredients for one cup (240 ml) are:

Basic Ingredients
1/4 cup (60 ml) Distilled Water
1/2 tsp. (2.5 ml) Xanthan Gum
Botanical Ingredients
2 Tbsp. (30 ml) Witch Hazel Water
2 Tbsp. (30 ml) Sage Tincture
1 Tbsp. (15 ml) Burdock Tincture
1/2 tsp. (2.5 ml) Provitamin B5
1/2 tsp. (2.5 ml) Vitamin C
Surfactants
3 Tbsp. (45 ml) Coco Betaine
3 Tbsp. (45 ml) Polyglucose
Essential Oils
15 drops Lavender
8 drops Sweet Orange
6 drops Tea Tree

Herbal Scalp Tonic For Oily Dandruff

To effectively reduce excessive sebum and scale production, it is advisable to apply this tonic on a daily basis. A rosemary decoction is used as the basic ingredient. Rosemary has a potent antiseptic activity, while Birch, and Burdock are antiinflammatory. The vitamins help to sustain normal cell regeneration. Since this tonic water does not contain lecithin or any oils, it should no longer be used when the scalp becomes defatted and dry. The ingredients for one half cup (120 ml) are:

Basic Ingredients
1/3 cup (80 ml) Rosemary Decoction
Botanical Ingredients
1 Tbsp. (15 ml) Burdock
1 Tbsp. (15 ml) Sage Tincture
1 Tbsp. (15 ml) Aloe Vera
1/4 tsp. (1.3 ml) Vitamin C
1/4 tsp. (1.3 ml) Vitamin E
1/4 tsp. (1.3 ml) Provitamin B5
1/8 tsp. (0.7 ml) Vitamin A
Essential Oils
5 drops Lemon
4 drops Tea Tree

Hair Conditioners

Dry hair lacks gloss and lustre, is harsh to touch, difficult to style, and is often subject to static electricity. This results from natural weathering, but it is particularly worsened by shampoos, which contain harsh and aggressive surfactants. Such hair is often totally devoid of sebum and desquamated scales. Hence, it needs to be conditioned to restore its manageability, softness, shine, and fullness. In addition, bad looking hair is most likely damaged, which some conditioners may be able to repair.

Soft, Shiny, and Healthy Hair

Conditioning agents are special surfactants, which fall into three different categories: film forming surfactants, protein-conjugated surfactants and cationic surfactants. Cationic surfactants, consisting of quaternary ammonium compounds (quats), function by neutralizing static electricity, which is caused by impaired hair cuticles. Since damaged hair shafts become negatively charged (anionic), the positively charged quats readily adhere to the hair and deposit a positively charged (cationic) film.

Film-forming conditioners are synthetic polymers, which are often attached to quats that coat the hair shaft and fill in the surface cuticle defects. Protein-based conditioners, which are also often quats, are combined with fragmented (hydrolyzed) proteins. When applied to the hair, these protein fragments penetrate the hair shaft and become linked with the proteins of the hair, particularly keratin. Thus, the damaged hair can be repaired by replacing lost proteins. Split ends become mended, and the hair regains its shine, softness, and manageability. It is notable, however, that these protective protein films will not remain attached at the hair cuticles forever. Natural weathering and shampooing will subsequently remove the conditioning agents. Thus, conditioners should be used regularly.

In my recipes, I have used a protein-based conditioner, which is briefly called collagen quat. Its full chemical name and special properties are further explained in the chapter about ingredients (page 73). Lecithin, honey, and an additional protein, such as soy protein, will further improve the conditioning effect. I have created three different conditioners for either normal, dry, or damaged hair. The latter should be used after waving, bleaching, or dyeing the hair, or after extensive sun exposure. All three formulas provide exclusive conditioners and should not be used as a shampoo. The basis of two of the conditioners is an emulsion consisting of oils, hot water, and an emulsifier. The procedure for preparing emulsion is described on page 18.

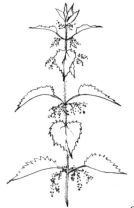

Stinging Nettle
(urtiga dioica)

Herbal Conditioner for Normal to Dry Hair

This conditioner will help to protect and strengthen the hair. It contains two different nourishing herbs and provitamin B5. Apply this conditioner to freshly washed, towel-dried hair and rinse it out after one minute (dry hair after three minutes). The hair will have maximum body, bounce, and fullness. It will be easy to style, and touchably beautiful. The ingredients for one half cup (120 ml) are:

Emulsion Basis
1 tsp. (5 ml) Almond Oil
1 tsp. (5 ml) Sorbitan Stearate
1/2 tsp. (2.5 ml) Polysorbate 60
1/3 cup. (80 ml) Hot Distilled Water
Botanical Ingredients
2 tsp. (10 ml) Aloe Vera
2 tsp. (10 ml) Stinging Nettle
Tincture
2 tsp. (10 ml) Lemon Juice
1/2 tsp. (2.5 ml) Soy Protein
1/2 tsp. (2.5 ml) Provitamin B5
1/4 tsp. (1.3 ml) Honey
1/4 tsp. (1.3 ml) Xanthan Gum
Surfactant
1/2 tsp. (2.5 ml) Collagen Quat
Essential Oils
5 drops Sandalwood
5 drops Rosemary
Preservative
10 drops Paraben/DiU

Vitamin Conditioner for Damaged Hair

A damaged hairshaft has disrupted cuticles, which render the hair porous and more susceptible to the effects of static electricity. However, the hair can be restored by the collagen fragments of the surfactant. Herbal tinctures, lecithin, and vitamins additionally nourish and moisturize the hair, preventing it from dehydrating. It will come alive with a healthy, shiny appearance. The ingredients for one half cup (120 ml) are:

Emulsion Basis
1 tsp. (5 ml) Jojoba Oil
1 tsp. (5 ml) Sorbitan Stearate
1/2 tsp. (2.5 ml) Polysorbate 60
1/2 tsp. (2.5 ml) Vitamin E
1/3 cup (80 ml) Hot Distilled Water
Botanical Ingredients
2 tsp. (10 ml) Stinging Nettle
Tincture
2 tsp. (10 ml) Calendula Tincture
2 tsp. (10 ml) Lemon Juice
1 tsp. (5 ml) Soy Protein
1 tsp. (5 ml) Provitamin B5
1/4 tsp. (1.3 ml) Lecithin
1/4 tsp. (1.3 ml) Xanthan Gum
1/8 tsp. (0.7 ml) Vitamin A
Surfactant
1 tsp. (5 ml) Collagen Quat
Essential Oils
7 drops Chamomile
7 drops Lavender
Preservative
10 drops Paraben/DiU

Herbal Rinse
For Dry Hair

Dry hair often lacks shine and produces electrical discharges when brushed or combed. Therefore, dry hair should be treated regularly with a refatting and moisturizing herbal rinse or conditioner. Use this hair rinse on towel-dried hair and do not wash it out. Vitamins, lecithin and herbs will get attached to the hairshaft and protect the hair from drying out. The ingredients for one half cup (120 ml) are:

Basic Ingredients
1/3 cup (80 ml) Distilled Water
Botanical Ingredients
1 Tbsp. (15 ml) Aloe Vera
1 Tbsp. (15 ml) Stinging Nettle Tincture
1 Tbsp. (15 ml) Chamomile Tincture
2 tsp. (10 ml) Lemon Juice
1/2 tsp. (2.5 ml) Soy Protein
1/2 tsp. (2.5 ml) Provitamin B5
1/2 tsp. (2.5 ml) Vitamin E
1/4 tsp. (1.3 ml) Lecithin
Emulsifier
1/4 tsp. (1.3 ml) Polysorbate 80
Surfactant
1/2 tsp. (2.5 ml) Collagen Quat
Essential Oils
6 drops Lavender
3 drops Ylang Ylang
Preservative
10 drops Paraben/DiU

Ingredients

Basic Ingredients

Distilled Water

Normal tap water is rich in mineral salts and metals such as calcium, magnesium, sodium, potassium, zinc, iron, aluminum, and others. The concentration of all these elements, in particular calcium, magnesium, and iron, determines the degree of hardness of the water. When used as drinking water, these salts are highly desirable. They are responsible for the richness and taste of the water and also for our health.

However, a high content of dissolved mineral salts, metals, and other impurities make the water unsuitable for many other purposes. Organic components, including proteins, sugars, and lipids may change their properties and lose their specific functions, when suspended in hard water. Moreover, mineral salts influence the acidity of water. Generally, the more minerals that are present, the more alkaline is the water. In cosmetic products, however, alkalinity is undesirable, since it reduces the viscosity of a solution and additionally impairs the acid mantle of the skin.

Therefore, when used in cosmetic applications, water is always demineralized. Removal of mineral salts is generally done by distillation or by passing the water through ion-absorbing compounds. Distillation means evaporation and subsequent condensation. In order to achieve top quality, self-made cosmetics, I strongly recommend the exclusive use of distilled water.

Plant Infusions, Teas

To achieve a herbal basis in cosmetic formulations, distilled water can be replaced by tea, which is also called plant infusion. They are easily produced by steeping plant leaves, ideally in a strainer, in hot water for a couple of minutes. For all recipes in this book, I encourage you to use your preferred tea or an infusion of your favorite garden plant. However, do not use tap water. Instead, use distilled water.

Plant Decoctions

Similar to plant infusions, decoctions can be used as the basic ingredients instead of distilled water. It is an easy, but effective method to extract different botanical components from plants. In contrast to infusions, the plants are boiled in water for a longer period of time (up to one hour), but at a lower temperature. Generally, decoctions are used primarily for hard botanical materials, such as roots, sticks, twigs, and barks. The extraction rate of the active ingredients is usually higher than that of infusions. Besides straining, it is advisable to pour the extract through a filter (e.g., coffee filters), since roots and barks often release small particles. Use distilled rather than tap water for preparing decoctions.

Xanthan Gum

Xanthan gum is a natural sugar (polysaccharide), which is derived from bacteria (xanthomonas campestris) and is used primarily as a thickener. It is a powder and is readily soluble upon stirring in water. Besides normal xanthan gum, there is also a pre-hydrated form available, which is more easily made dispersible by reducing the tendency to form lumps. By absorbing moisture, xanthan gum swells considerably and forms a viscous liquid. Dependent upon the concentration, xanthan gum is capable of turning every hydrous liquid into a highly viscous gel. To achieve a homogenous solution, xanthan gum should be mixed thoroughly with an electric mixer. Xanthan gum can be stored at room temperature.

Sheabutter
(butyrospermum parkii)

Sheabutter is a plant fat extracted from plum-like nuts, which grow on large tropic trees in West Africa. The oil is widely used by African natives. Due to the high content of unsaponifiable and cinnamic esters, sheabutter has excellent skin care properties. It moisturizes, refats, and protects effectively from solar radiation. Sheabutter contains allantoin, vitamin A and E, which promote wound healing and provide a potent antioxidant effect. Similar to common cooking butter, sheabutter will spoil at room temperature and thus needs to be stored refrigerated.

Plant Distillates

Plant distillates are a by-product of the steam distillation in the purification process of essential oils. Plant distillates are clear and highly purified. Generally, they have similar properties as essential oils, but in much less concentration. Plant distillates make excellent facial splashes and can be used undiluted. They are mostly utilized for cleansing lotions and tonic waters. However, dependent upon the herb used for a distillate, the effects on the skin will vary considerably. Distillates can be combined to create a desired scent or to intensify a certain effect. Though many different kinds of distillates are available, I have chosen the three most common.

Orange Flower Water

Orange flower water produces mild antiseptic and antiinflammatory reaction and provides for a soothing and astringent effect on the skin. It is suitable for all skin types, particularly for sensitive and aging skin. The fundamental citric ingredient of oranges gives a very refreshing feeling on the skin. When combined with rose water, its soothing effect is even more appreciated.

Rose Water

Because of its wonderful and intense scent of roses, rose water is often used to provide perfume for skin and hair preparations. However, it is also well-known to relieve dryness and roughness, and to reduce the fragility of capillaries in aging skin. Due to its excellent soothing properties, rose water is an indispensable ingredient for sensitive skin.

Witch Hazel Water

Witch hazel water provides many beneficial effects. It reduces itching and irritations of the skin, and is a very valuable ingredient in antiacneic cleansing lotions. Along with aloe vera, witch hazel water is one of the most important botanical agents with antiinflammatory and healing benefits. It is thus a very effective component in the treatment of sun-irritated or sunburnt skin. Witch hazel is particularly effective when combined with aloe vera.

Tinctures and Plant Extracts

Similar to plant infusions and decoctions, tinctures and plant extracts, which are also called fluid extracts, are liquids containing soluble ingredients, that are drawn from the cells of a plant. However, both tinctures and plant extracts are cold extractions, which are made by steeping herbs in alcoholic solutions. The difference between tinctures and plant extracts lies in their strength. Fluid extracts consist of one part solvent and one part herb, whereas tinctures typically contain one part herb and five to ten parts solvent. The concentration of the alcohol will vary, but its addition is crucial, since it allows the fat-soluble substances of a plant to be extracted. Thus, tinctures and fluid extracts are comparable to essential oils with regard to their medicinal properties.

Both tinctures and plant extracts are commercially available. Before using a commercial product, take care to notice whether it is a fluid extract or a tincture. Because all recipes are calculated for tinctures, fluid extracts need to be diluted about five times with distilled water.

However, you can save a lot of money by processing them yourself. The procedure is very easy. Ideally, the herbs are initially dried and chopped, but you can also use fresh plants. Conveniently, many health and herb stores offer different kinds of herbs, which are already in powdered form. Place these herbs in a glass jar, which has a tightly fitting lid and add distilled water and alcohol. You may use purified ethyl alcohol, but grain alcohol such as vodka or dry gin, works just as well. Make sure that the herbs are covered by the liquid and allow them to steep for at least two weeks. The mixture can then be strained through a cheesecloth and placed in a dark glass bottle. Do not forget to put a label on it with the date and the plant name. Generally, tinctures have a shelf life of up to two years. The following recipe provides a herbal tincture of about one cup.

1. Place 2 oz. (60 grams) of herbs in a glass jar.
When using fresh herbs, you can add more.

2. Add ½ cup (120 ml) of grain alcohol, such as vodka or dry gin.
Ethyl alcohol is used at a concentration of 50%.
Important: do not use rubbing alcohol (isopropyl alcohol).

3. Add ½ cup (120 ml) of distilled water and make sure
that the herbs are covered by the liquid.

4. Allow the mixture to steep for at least two weeks and shake
the jar regularly to keep the herbs from settling.

5. Press the mixture thoroughly through several layers of
cheesecloth and place the extract in a dark glass bottle.

Aloe Vera
(aloe barbadensis, aloe vulgaris)

Aloe vera is a lily-like plant with potent healing properties. Due to its high amount of vitamin E and C, it has potent antioxidant and antiinflammatory properties. It is, therefore, a valuable ingredient for the treatment of inflamed and irritated skin, including sunburns, eczema, and contact dermatitis. Aloe vera can be clinically used for the treatment of frostbites and wounds. Also, the fresh juice of the plant is often used as first aid for minor burns and wounds. In addition, aloe vera has good moisturizing, soothing, and antiitching benefits. Cosmetics which contain aloe vera will spoil less due to the antibacterial and antifungal properties. Aloe vera can be used as undiluted fresh plant juice (gel), as a concentrate, or as a diluted liquid (contains at least 50% of plant juice). In my recipes, I always use undiluted plant juice.

Birch
(betula pendula)

Birch extracts and tinctures are made from the bark, the leaves, and the juice of the tree. Due to its stimulating effect on cell growth, it is primarily used in preparations to guard against hair loss. Birch has also been shown to have antiseptic activity and is thus recommended for acneic skin. In many preparations, birch is used as an astringent agent.

Burdock
(arctium lappa)

The active ingredients of burdock are extracted primarily from the roots and seeds of the plant. They are well-known for their potent healing power. Similar to birch, burdock stimulates cell growth and has antiinflammatory properties. It is very valuable in the treatment of dandruff, hair loss, inflamed skin, and acne.

Chamomile
(matricaria chamomilla/recutica and chamaemelum nobile)

There are basically two chamomile plants which are useful for skin and hair care products: the German chamomile (matricaria chamomilla/recutica) and the Roman chamomile (chamaemelum nobile). Both have daisy-like white and yellow heads, but the flowers of the German chamomile are smaller and smell different. The dried and powdered flowers from both plants are used for extracts, tinctures and teas. Because of their potent antiinflammatory properties, chamomile extracts are effective when used as a poultice to treat swellings and pain. In cosmetics and ointments, chamomile is widely utilized to soothe irritated skin, particularly dry and sensitive skin. In addition, chamomile extracts and tinctures are often used in hair shampoos and rinses for blonde hair to retain its natural color. The coloring agent is known as apigenin.

Comfrey
(symphytum officinale)

One of the major active ingredients of comfrey is allantoin. It is extracted from the leaves as well as from the flowering top. Allantoin has potent soothing and regenerating effects and is used in many dermatological formulations for the treatment of psoriasis, skin ulcers, burns, and wounds.

Echinacea, Purple Coneflower
(echinacea angustifolia)

Echinacea is one of the most widely used botanical products. Native Americans have for a long time had extensive knowledge about the medicinal use of the numerous echinacea species, which are found in the Midwest of North America. In particular, the roots and rhizomes of echinacea angustifolia have excellent regenerative and antiinflammatory properties. Similar to comfrey, it can be clinically applied to treat different skin diseases.

Ginseng
(panax ginseng)

Ginseng has long been considered as a universal remedy in Asian medicine. It is processed from the roots, which require as much as six years of cultivation to reach maturity. When used internally, ginseng has been reported to have beneficial effects on blood pressure, blood sugar, metabolism, and some believe it can prolong life. Likewise, when applied to the skin, ginseng enhances the cellular function and acts as a prophylaxis against aging of the skin. In many studies, ginseng has been shown to lengthen the life span of skin cells and stimulate their proliferation. Consequently, ginseng is often used in anti-wrinkle creams.

Gotu Kola
(centella asiatica)

Gotu kola is a perennial plant, which is native to Continental Asia, the South Pacific, and Africa. Dependent upon the climate, the plant can look very different. Gotu kola has remarkable wound healing properties. It is often used for burns, skin ulcers, and different kinds of wounds. In addition, some believe it can stimulate hair growth.

Marigold, Calendula
(Calendula officinalis)

Marigolds are seasonal plants and grow everywhere. Their extracts and tinctures are made from the dried, bright yellow flowers. Marigold has long been known as a healing remedy. In many skin formulations, it is a basic ingredient for the treatment of rashes, irritations, acne, burns, and other inflammations.

Marsh Mallow, Althea
(radix althaea)

The name of this plant is based on its healing property. In Greek, althea means "healing." Similar to aloe vera, the extracts and tinctures of althea have excellent antiinflammatory and regenerative effects. It is thus very valuable in after-sun formulations. Althea is also moisturizing, astringent, and soothing.

Plantain
(plantago major)

Plantain is a small weed and grows everywhere. Its leaves and seeds are known to have healing properties. When applied to the skin, plantain extracts will soothe and soften the skin. It is also often used for inflammations, such as stings and sunburns.

Sage
(salvia officinalis)

Sage extract and tincture are antiseptic, astringent, and reduces perspiration. Sage is an excellent ingredient in anti-dandruff formulations, such as shampoos or tonic waters. It also reduces itching and soothes skin irritations. Sage is believed to be capable of restoring the color of graying hair.

St. John's Wort
(hypericum perforatum)

St. John's wort grows all over the world and has been used for centuries as a universal remedy. Extracts and tinctures of this plant are made from the seeds and from the bright yellow flowers. Due to its antiseptic and antiinflammatory properties, St. John's wort is a very valuable ingredient in formulations for burns, acne, and irritated skin. It has also been found to help with healing of wounds.

Stinging Nettles
(urtiga dioica)

When grown in the back yard, stinging nettles are often not very welcome. However, they are very useful plants, which contain many healthy ingredients, primarily vitamins. Extracts of the roots and leaves of stinging nettles are known to improve the microcirculation in the skin. It is, therefore, often used in scalp tonic to treat hair loss and dandruff. In addition, it has a good conditioning effect and is thus very valuable in hair preparations. Stinging nettle is also effective against itching.

Witch Hazel
(hamamelis virginiana)

Witch hazel is a small tree growing throughout North America. It flowers in the fall. Extracts are made from dry leaves, barks, and twigs. Besides its potent antiinflammatory properties, witch hazel also has soothing and astringent qualities. It is, therefore, widely used in after-sun or after-shave formulations. Commercially, witch hazel is available as a distillate with or without alcohol.

Plant Oils

Almond Oil

Almond oil, which is a kernel oil, is obtained from the ripe seed of the small sweet almond that is grown in Southern Europe. Its purification and application have been known for hundreds of years. The oil is very mild and soothing. It leaves the skin soft and smooth. Almond oil has a pleasant, slightly sweet fragrance, which gives the oil a very special character.

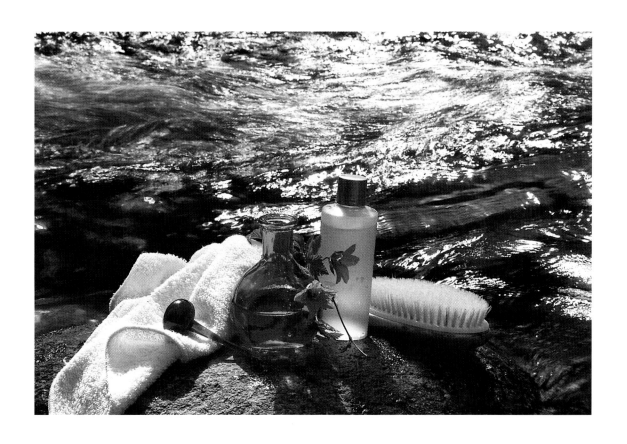

Bathing with precious, scented oils is a wonderful experience
for mind and body

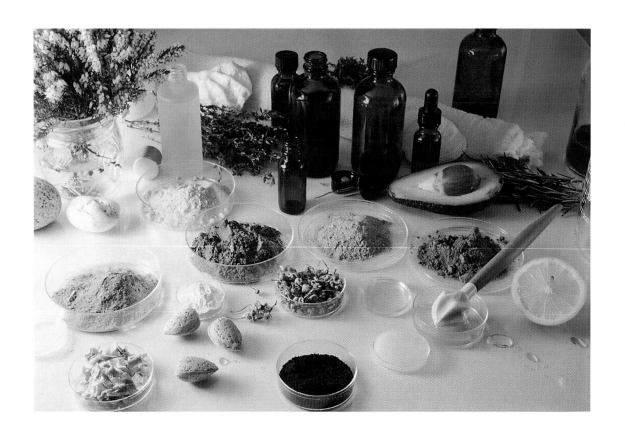

Creating your own cosmetics allows you to choose from
a broad selection of many different ingredients

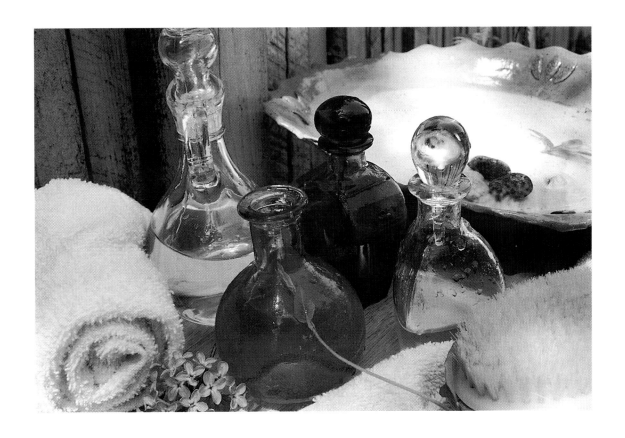

Plant oils are used as basic ingredients for creams, lotions, and bath oils, and provide many good nourishing and regenerating benefits

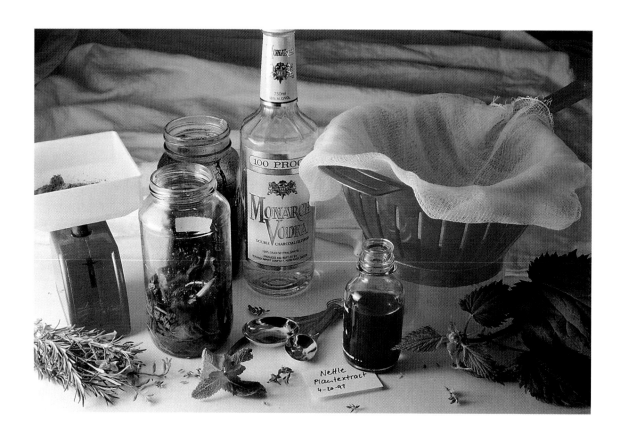

Herbal tinctures are easily self-made
from plants, water, and alcohol

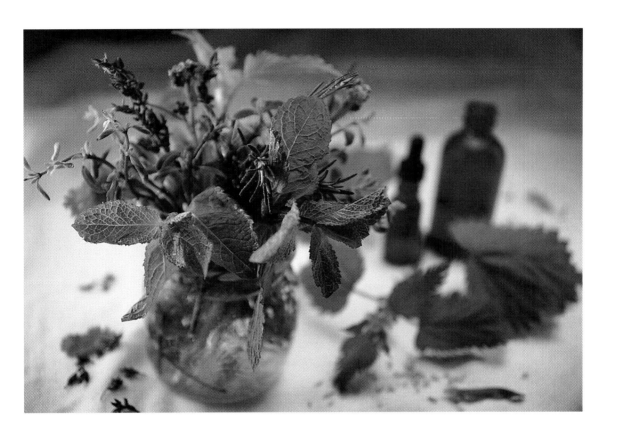

Essential oils are the aromatic contents of plants and are very valuable ingredients based on their intense scent and numerous therapeutic properties

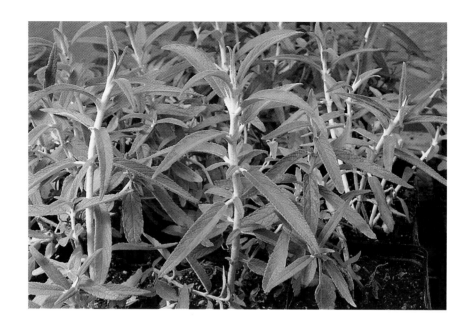

Sage
(salvia officinalis)

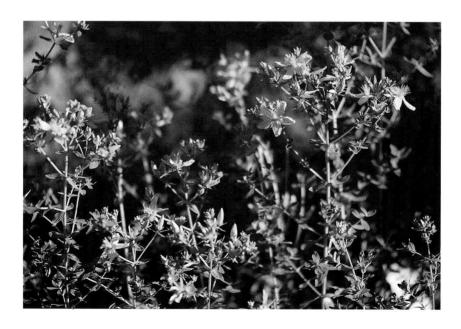

St. John's Wort
(hypericum perforatum)

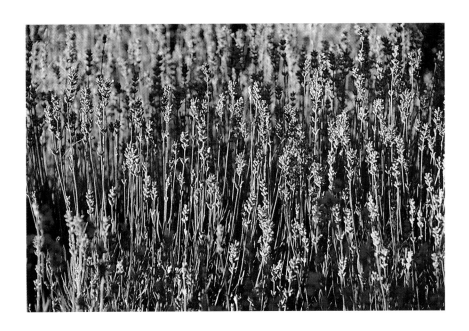

Lavender
(lavendula officinalis)

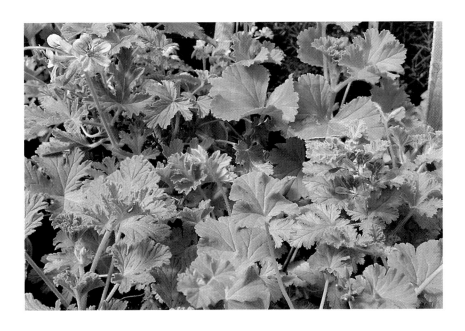

Rose Geranium
(pelargonium roseum)

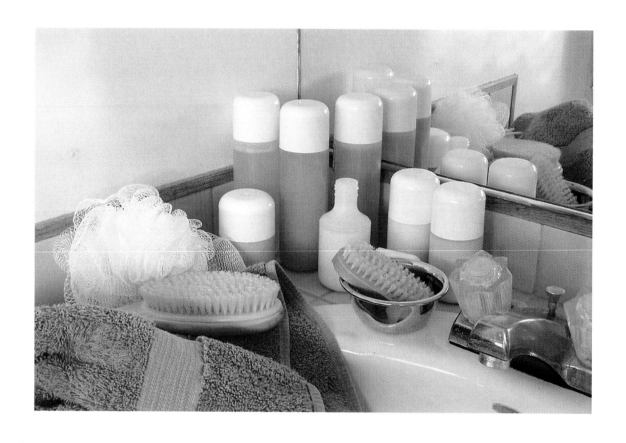

Your personal cosmetic line will consist of a complete set of
modern, natural body care products

Apricot Kernel Oil

Similar to sweet almond oil, apricot oil is also a kernel oil and has similar properties. However, when applied to the skin, it is less greasy than almond oil and is thus especially suited for formulations applied to the face. The skin can be softened and gently refatted without producing an oily sheen.

Avocado Oil

Avocado fruit is not only delicious, but is also very healthy, since it contains many unsaturated fatty acids. The unprocessed oil of the fruit is also a rich source of lecithin, vitamin E and different vitamins of the B-complex. On skin and hair, avocado oil provides many good nourishing and regenerating benefits.

Calendula Oil (Marigold)

This seasonal herb (calendula officinalis) is well-known for its healing powers. The oil is derived from the bright yellow flowers. It is a very valuable ingredient for different kinds of skin problems, including rough skin, diaper rash, eczema, and inflammations. It is thus especially suited for skin care formulations for sensitive skin or baby skin.

Jojoba Oil

This oil is obtained from the nut-like seed of the jojoba tree (pronounced as "ho-ho-ba") that grows in the dry and warm climate of subtropical deserts. The oil is in fact a wax. It becomes a liquid at room temperature, but will quickly turn waxy when stored in the refrigerator. Unlike other vegetable oils, jojoba oil does not spoil, which suggests the presence of potent antibacterial substances. When applied to the skin, it has a soothing effect and protects the skin from solar radiation. It is also helpful for the treatment of acne. Due to its similar biochemical properties, jojoba oil has largely replaced sperm whale oil (spermaceti oil). Sperm whale oil was widely used by the cosmetic industry, when whale hunting was more common. However, sperm whale oil is in no way any better than jojoba oil.

Soybean Oil

Soybean oil is extracted from the seeds of soy plants, which grow primarily in the Far East, and also in the Midwest of the USA. It contains many unsaturated fatty acids, proteins, lecithin, and vitamin E. Due to this natural richness, it is often refined to gain proteins and lecithin. Unprocessed soybean oil is a very nourishing oil for the skin and hair, which is useful for many preparations.

Wheat Germ Oil

Wheat germ oil is a rich source of lecithin and vitamins E, A and D. Besides its nourishing effect, it is well-known for its antiaging properties. This is primarily due to the antioxidant activity of vitamin E, which neutralizes the cell-damaging effects of free radicals. Radicals are oxygen products, which are released from disturbed skin cells. They alter the regeneration of tissue and induce premature skin aging. Thus, wheat germ oil is often utilized in anti-wrinkle creams.

Other Plant Oils

Basically, most plant oils are appropriate for cosmetic skin and hair care formulations. For instance, safflower oil, sesame oil, corn oil, olive oil, and sunflower oil are all very useful. Hence, dependent upon your preferences, you may utilize any of these other plant oils. For the recipes in this book, I have chosen oils, which are all known for their beneficial effects for the skin.

However, I do not recommend using mineral oils. These are made from highly refined petroleum and do not contain any botanical ingredients. They form a shiny film on the skin, rather than penetrate the surface. Moreover, mineral oils have often been found to induce allergic reactions. However, despite these disadvantages, mineral oils are still widely used in commercial cosmetics.

Oils can spoil in a relatively short period of time. Make sure that the oils are fresh when bought, and do not store them for more than a couple of weeks after having opened the bottle. Spoiling can be reduced by the addition of a small amount of vitamin E (see the following).

Vitamins

Vitamin A (retinol)

Vitamin A is one of four fat-soluble vitamins. Besides its important function as a visual pigment for the eyes, vitamin A is an indispensable natural agent for the normal growth and development of cells. It plays an important part in the generation of the horny layer of the skin (keratinization). Its drawback is that this can lead to excessive horn formation (hyperkeratosis). The addition of vitamin A to skin care products helps to maintain the normal regeneration and metabolism of the tissue. Since it is not soluble in water, vitamin A is often dissolved in a plant oil. It should be stored refrigerated and protected from the light.

Vitamin E (tocopherol)

Similar to vitamin A, vitamin E is also fat-soluble. It is generally found in plant oils. Vitamin E is well-known to exert potent antiinflammatory and antioxidant activities. Antioxidants are agents, which are able to neutralize free radicals, that are highly reactive, tissue-damaging oxygen derivatives released from disturbed cells. Such radicals have been found to occur in many diseases. Potent antioxidants, however, such as vitamin E, effectively alleviate such pathologic processes.

Vitamin E penetrates deep into the skin and acts as a potent moisturizing and antiinflammatory agent. It also protects against UV radiation, and has good antiaging properties. Vitamin E is available in different forms. I prefer vitamin E acetate, since it is more stable than other forms and is easy to use. It is clear, viscous, odorless, and can be added directly to the formulas. By adding some drops to plant oils you can effectively reduce spoiling. Vitamin E should be stored refrigerated and protected from the light.

Vitamin C (ascorbic acid)

Vitamin C is water-soluble. It occurs naturally in large amounts in citric fruits, such as lemons, oranges, or grapefruit. Vitamin C is essential for the normal growth of bones and the maintenance of healthy skin. Depletion of vitamin C significantly impairs the production of collagen in the skin.

Similar to vitamin E, vitamin C is a potent antioxidant, which is capable of diminishing the tissue damaging effects of free oxygen radicals. Since such radicals have been found to be involved in many different diseases, both vitamin C and E are currently being tested in several clinical studies. For instance, it has been demonstrated that vitamin C is able to promote healing of wounds and effectively protect the skin from the effects of UV radiation. Due to its antibacterial properties, vitamin C can also reduce spoiling in cosmetic products. Vitamin C is a white powder that darkens upon exposure to air.

Provitamin B5 (panthenol)

Panthenol, which is also called pantothenic acid, is a precursor of vitamin B5 and is rapidly metabolized to an active vitamin B5 after absorption. Similar to all vitamins of the B-complex, provitamin B5 is water-soluble. It sustains and promotes the growth of many cell types. When applied to the skin, provitamin B5 provides protection from the radiation of the sun, and helps to regenerate irritated or aging skin. In addition, provitamin B5 accumulates humidity in the tissue, which prevents the skin from dehydrating and chapping. It also has potent antiinflammatory properties. In hair preparations, provitamin B5 effectively moisturizes, which gives the hair fullness and elasticity. Provitamin B5 is viscous and clear. It should be stored in the refrigerator.

Other Botanical Ingredients

Proteins

As well as sugars and lipids, proteins are the basic constituents of all living organisms. Each cell synthesizes hundreds of different proteins. Skin cells, in particular, produce large amounts of collagen, elastin, and keratin. Collagen and elastin form the major components of the connective tissue of the skin. Collagen is fibrous and rigid, while elastin is elastic and flexible. Both sustain many important functions in the skin, such as stability, elasticity, humidity and protection. Keratin is the major component of hair and nails, and forms the horny layers of the skin. If the production of these tissue proteins is impaired, this can lead to thin, fragile, paper-like skin, similar to that which normally occurs in aging skin.

Proteins have long been used as excellent humectants in cosmetics. When applied to the skin, proteins will attach to the outer cell layer, forming a soft, protective, and moisturizing film. However, they cannot penetrate the horny layer of the skin, even when chemically reduced to small fractions (hydrolysation). Proteins are mostly used as hydrolysates in cosmetics, in order to increase their solubility. However, their tendency to gelatinization can be utilized to augment the viscosity of a solution. Thus, proteins can be used as natural thickeners.

There are many different kinds of purified proteins, mostly hydrolysates, on the market. While collagen, elastin, and keratin are most common, other proteins derived from wheat, soybeans, vegetables, and marine plants, are also suitable. In my recipes, proteins are added either as collagen-conjugated surfactants or as hydrolyzed soy protein.

Honey

Honey is a rich source of not only different natural sugars (poly- and monosaccharides), but also many proteins. In shampoos, honey is well-known as a valuable conditioner. It lubricates the hair and gives it fullness and volume. While depositing a soft glossy film, honey has effective soothing and emollient effects on the skin.

Lecithin

Lecithin is a mixture of phospholipids, which form the membrane of human, animal, and plant cells. This phospholipid coat is arranged as a double layer, which is very compact, but is still permeable for small molecules. Phospholipids consist of two lipophilic fatty tails and a hydrophilic phosphate group. Due to this unique structure, lecithin is able to mix fat and water, and can be used as a natural emulsifier.

Lecithin is mainly extracted from soybeans and egg yolks and appears brown and yellowish in color. However, pure lecithin is not suitable as a cosmetic emulsifier, and needs more processing. When purchasing lecithin, it is thus important to ask for lecithin, which is capable of being used as a cosmetic emulsifier. For purposes other than emulsifying, one can also use unprocessed lecithin. Some lecithins tend to form lumps in water. This can be avoided by dissolving lecithin in a small amount of grain alcohol, such as vodka or dry gin. When applied to the skin, lecithin readily penetrates the horny layer, entering deeply into the tissue. It effectively acts as an emollient, moisturizer, and a regenerating agent.

Lemon Juice

Normal skin is slightly acid. Acidity and alkalinity is expressed as a pH-value ranging from 1 (most acid) to 14 (most alkaline). The skin has a value of 5 to 6 and is thus close to the neutral value of pH 7. It has been shown that the use of alkaline cosmetic products can destroy the acid mantle of the skin. This can cause increased irritability of the skin, which promotes the occurrence of allergies and inflammations. Cosmetics should, therefore, be neutral or slightly acid. Lemon juice, with its strong, natural acidity, is ideal to keep cosmetic formulations more acidic. Since all recipes are already neutral or only slightly alkaline, a small amount should be sufficient.

Surfactants

Although water is most effective for cleansing, it is not able to remove fatty particles from the skin. Therefore, it is necessary to add substances, which are capable of being mixed with the fatty mantle of the skin. Such cleansing agents are called surface-active agents or for short, surfactants. They act at the surface between fat and water, thereby forming foam. When surfactants are applied to the skin, they allow fatty dirt to be suspended in water. The particles are then easily removed by rubbing and rinsing with water.

One of the most potent and widely used surfactants is soap. However, it contains a high concentration of skin irritating salts, is alkaline, is always solid and is not useful for any other purposes than cleansing. Modern cleansing agents, called syndets or liquid soaps, overcome these disadvantages and provide many additional benefits. They are mostly neutral and are more convenient and hygienic, because they are liquid and thus are more easily dispensable. Moreover, they are also applicable as a conditioner, an emulsifier, an emollient, a viscosifier, or a humectant. Hence, modern liquid soaps are highly sophisticated synthetic products. However, they are not completely synthetic. The major constituents, which are the fatty acids, are derived from natural oils.

Not all surfactants are mild. Many commercial, cosmetic products contain cheap surfactants, which often can cause eye and skin irritations or allergies. Based on numerous dermatological studies, the following surfactants have been found to be problematic: sodium lauryl sulfate, sodium laureth sulfate, disodium laureth sulfate, benzalkonium chloride, cocamido DEA, and lauramido DEA. A recent report has shown that the irritancy of surfactants is also dependent on the water temperature. Showering at temperatures above 104°F (40°C) significantly increases the occurrence of skin irritations induced by surfactants.

For my recipes, I have selected four different surfactants, which are known to be very mild. They are exclusively synthesized from natural products, are neutral or slightly acidic, and contain very low amounts of salts. The names of the surfactants used in these recipes are abbreviations. Their full chemical names are listed below. Usually, surfactants also have tradenames, which can vary dependent upon the company. Thus, surfactants can be ordered by their chemical or also by their tradename.

Coco Betaine
(cocoamidopropyl betaine)

This surfactant is made from coconut oil. Since the molecule is electrochemically neutral, it belongs to the group of amphoteric surfactants, which are generally very mild. It has cleansing, emulsifying, foaming, and also conditioning properties. The antistatic effect prevents the hair from becoming negatively charged and tangled after washing ("fly away" hair). The effects of coco betaine is further increased by the combination of non-ionic surfactants, such as coco collagen and polyglucose. Coco betaine is biodegradable.

Coco Collagen
(potassium coco hydrolyzed collagen)

This surfactant is composed of hydrolyzed proteins (collagen) and fatty acids derived from coconut oil. It belongs to the group of non-ionic surfactants, since it does not have an electrochemical charge. It has cleansing, thickening, emulsifying, and emollient effects. Coco collagen is very mild. It does not irritate either skin, hair, nor eyes. When used in combination with amphoteric surfactants, such as coco betaine, the effects of both surfactants are reinforced. Coco collagen is often used to complete a recipe with proteins. It is also biodegradable.

Polyglucose
(decyl polyglucose)

Decyl polyglucose is synthesized from natural sugars (polyglycosides) and fatty acids. As coco collagen, it is a non-ionic surfactant and thus has similar properties. It can be used as a primary surfactant or also as a secondary agent to further improve the cleansing and emulsifying effects of other surfactants. Generally, non-ionic surfactants, consisting of natural sugar components, are considered to be exceptionally mild. Polyglucose is biodegradable.

Collagen Quat
(lauryl dimonium hydrolyzed collagen)

Due to a positive electrochemical charge, collagen quat belongs to the group of cationic surfactants. Such surfactants are often simply called "quats," since they contain a quaternary ammonium group. The most important property of quats is their excellent hair conditioning effect. Collagen quat contains hydrolyzed collagen, which becomes attached to the hair cuticles and forms a protective layer. This softens and repairs the cuticles of the hair and provides for fullness, shine, and gloss. It reduces "fly away" hair and prevents the hair from getting tangled. Collagen quat is very mild and biodegradable.

Emulsifiers

Similar to surfactants, emulsifiers are substances, which are able to mix oil with water. Both have similar chemical structure, which consists of a lipophilic tail and a hydrophilic head. Emulsifiers, however, have the capability to combine oil and water to a very stable, permanent solution, which is called an emulsion. While most emulsifiers consist of one or two fatty acids, which are attached to a glycerin molecule, there are numerous chemically different emulsifiers with very similar properties.

There are also some natural emulsifiers such as lecithin and algae derivatives. However, they usually have to be chemically modified to achieve an emulsifying effect, which is sufficient for cosmetic purposes. Since emulsifiers are primarily utilized for creams and ointments, I am not going to discuss any further the different cosmetic emulsifiers and their properties. All three emulsifiers which I have used in some of the recipes in this book, are described below.

Sorbitan Stearate

Sorbitan stearate belongs to the group of sorbitan esters. It is composed of stearate, a fatty acid, and sorbitol, a natural sugar. Sorbitol occurs naturally in different fruits, particularly in the berries of the mountain ash, and is used as a sugar substitute. Sorbitan stearate is available as powder or flakes. It acts as thickener and emulsifier, particularly in combination with polyoxyethylated sorbitan esters, such as polysorbate 60 and polysorbate 80.

Polysorbate 60
(polyoxyethylene sorbitan monostearate)

As sorbitan stearate, polysorbate 60 is also a sorbitan ester, composed of stearate and sorbitol, but is supplemented with polyoxyethylene. This increases the capability to form emulsions. When combined with sorbitan stearate, polysorbate 60 forms a very stable emulsion. It is thus used primarily as co-emulsifier. Polysorbate 60 is semi-solid and waxy.

Polysorbate 80
(polyoxyethylene sorbitan monooleate)

Originally, polysorbate 80 was used essentially as a food emulsifier. It is also a polyoxyethylated sorbitan ester, but contains oleate as fatty acid, instead of stearate. Polysorbate 80 is very mild, as are all sorbitol-based emulsifiers. No toxicity is known to be present. In cosmetic formulations, polysorbate 80 helps to stabilize essential oils and fat soluble vitamins. In addition, polysorbate 80 is very useful in bath oils to achieve a better dispersion. Polysorbate 80 is liquid and has a sweet caramel-like odor.

Essential Oils

The scent or "essence" of a plant is based on its content of different oils, which constantly evaporate into the air. Such botanical volatile oils are called essential oils, which represent the odoriferous principles of a plant. They can be found in flowers, leaves, fruit peel, bark, wood, root, or resin of a plant. The production of essential oils is not quite that easy. It may be achieved by either mechanical extraction of the botanical material, or by distillation by steamed water. Dependent upon the content of volatile oils in a plant and the necessity of further purification steps, the extraction process of essential oils and consequently their price can vary considerably. Furthermore, the quality and aromatic intensity of an oil may change dependent upon the season of harvesting the plants.

Certain volatile oils are not obtained by distillation, but are extracted by organic solvents. Such oils are waxlike substances called **concretes**. They are primarily prepared from the flowers, leaves, and barks. Concretes are more concentrated than essential oils. Jasmine is an example. When a concrete is further processed by a second solvent extraction with alcohol, the unwanted wax is removed and the extract becomes a viscous liquid called **absolute**.

It has been shown that stimulation of the olfactory sense may greatly influence mind and body. This effect is utilized systematically in the aromatherapy. Unfortunately, this kind of therapy is not yet regularly applied in the clinical routine. However, essential oils are widely used as potent active ingredients in skin care products. Consisting of small molecules, essential oils are able to penetrate the skin without leaving oily residues. The recommended concentration is about 1 to 3% dependent upon the intensity of the aroma. An accurate dosage is achieved by a medicinal dropper. Many oils have also antiseptic activity and can be used as natural preservatives.

Bergamot
(citrus bergamia)

This oil is extracted by cold extraction of the fresh peel of the orange-like bergamot fruit. Due to its fruity-sweet citrus aroma, it is widely used in soaps and perfumes. It is a valuable ingredient for preparations to treat acne, oily skin and greasy hair. Bergamot oil should not be applied to sun-exposed skin, because it may cause irreversible hyperpigmentations (berloque dermatitis).

Cajeput
(melaleuca leucadendron)

Cajeput essential oil is obtained by steam distillation from fresh leaves and twigs. It has a mild, camphor-like scent with a fruity character. Cajeput oil is astringent and is effective for treating muscle sores.

German or Blue Chamomile
(matricaria chamomilla/recutica)

This essential oil is extracted from the flower heads of the German chamomile. It is pale blue due to the presence of azulene. It also contains alpha-bisabolol, which is thought to be mainly responsible for the strong antiinflammatory and antispasmodic effects of the oil. Chamomile has a herbaceous scent and has excellent soothing effects. It has been used successfully in the treatment of rashes, dermatitis, eczema, and acne. Roman chamomile (chamaemelum nobile) has similar but less pronounced effects, probably due to the lower concentration of azulene and alpha-bisabolol.

Clary Sage
(salvia sclarea)

The essential oil of clary sage is obtained by steam distillation from the flowering tops and leaves of the plant. It has a deep, warm, and sweet aroma with a refreshing and stimulating effect. When used on the skin, clary sage feels very soothing, relaxing, and acts effectively against dandruff and oily skin. When used as warm compresses or massage oils, it softens cramps and sores. Clary sage is also available as a concrete.

Eucalyptus
(eucalyptus globulus)

Eucalyptus species are evergreen trees, from which the leaves and twigs are used to extract the essential oil. It is produced by steam distillation. Eucalyptus is well-known for the relief of colds and muscular aches. It has potent antiinflammatory properties, which are useful against insect bites and minor skin infections.

Grapefruit
(citrus paradisi)

Grapefruit essential oil is extracted from the peel of the grapefruit by cold extraction. It has a sweet aroma along with a refreshing soothing effect. Grapefruit essential oil is often used for headaches. Similar to rose geranium, it has antiseptic properties and is thus a valuable ingredient in preparations for treating acne and oily skin. Grapefruit oil has been suggested as promoting hair growth.

Jasmine
(jasminum grandiflorum)

Jasmine oil is produced by solvent extraction and is thus available as a concrete or also as an absolute. It has an intense, sweet, floral scent and is widely used in perfumes and skin care products. Jasmine helps to relieve stress and nervous exhaustion and can also be used as an aphrodisiac. It is suitable for all skin types, but especially for dry and sensitive skin. Jasmine is one of the most expensive oils.

Juniper Berry
(junipers communis)

This essential oil is extracted by steam distillation. It has a deep, woody odor with a balsamic character. Juniper has antiseptic and antispasmodic properties and is helpful against acne, oily skin, and also hair loss. When added to bath oils, the scent of juniper has a relaxing effect.

Lavender
(lavendula officinalis)

When used as a traditional folklore remedy, the characteristic, sweet, floral-herbaceous scent of lavender is familiar to most people. Lavender is used as an effective ingredient for treating different skin affections, such as eczema, acne, infections, sunburns, oily scalp, dandruff, dry and sensitive skin, and insect bites. Moreover, it is suggested as being an effective insect repellent. The scent of lavender has a relaxing and sedative effect. Lavender oil is available as essential oil, concrete, or also as an absolute.

Lemon
(citrus limon)

Lemon oil is produced by cold extraction of the fresh outer peel. It smells very refreshing and stimulating. Lemon oil is antiseptic and is very effective against seborrhea and skin impurities. It is thus often used in hair preparations to treat dandruff and seborrhea. Similar to bergamot oil, lemon oil should not be used on sun-exposed skin. It may cause irreversible hyperpigmentations.

Lemon Balm
(melissa officinalis)

Lemon balm oil is extracted by steam distillation from the leaves and flowers of the lemon balm bush. It has long been used as an all-purpose medicinal herb. In particular, it can be used to treat insect bites and minor skin inflammations.

Marjoram
(origanum marjorana)

Marjoram is a traditional kitchen herb, which has a warm, woody, and spicy odor. This essential oil is produced by steam distillation of the dried flowering herb. Marjoram has various healing properties. It is known to soften cramps, relieve muscular aches, assist to heal wounds, and help to cure colds and coughs. The scent has a relaxing effect.

Neroli or Orange Blossom
(citrus aurantium)

For hundreds of years, the white freshly picked flowers of the orange blossom have been utilized for cosmetic purposes. Available as an essential oil, concrete, or also absolute, the oil has a warm, floral–sweet scent. It has a relaxing and soothing effect, which is ideal in formulations for sensitive or irritated skin. It is also used for treating dandruff. Neroli oil is one of the most expensive oils on the market.

Palmarosa
(cymbopogon martinii)

Because of its similar scent to rose geranium, palmarosa oil is also known as Indian or Turkish geranium oil. However, it is not derived from geranium plants, but from the family of graminaceae. The essential oil is extracted from the fragrant leaves of the plant-grass. The scent is sweet, floral, and slightly rosy. Palmarosa oil is used for acne, sores, skin infections, and seborrhea.

Patchouli
(pogostemon cablin)

Patchouli is a bushy herb up to three feet high and grows in many regions of Asia. This essential oil is produced by steam distillation of dried and fermented leaves. Patchouli oil has a rich, herbaceous, earthy aroma and is extensively used as a basic fragrance in cosmetic products. Due to its antiinflammatory properties, it is effective in the treatment of acne and dandruff. In China, patchouli is widely used as a folk remedy to treat colds, headaches, nausea, and vomiting.

Peppermint
(mentha piperita)

The strong, penetrating, minty odor of peppermint is probably due to it being the most popular scent of all plants. Its active ingredient, menthol, has a cooling, refreshing effect. In folk medicine, peppermint is often used in steam baths to help with coughs and colds. When applied to the skin, peppermint is very effective to help against itching, inflammations, swellings, and pain. It is also antiseptic and astringent. Peppermint essential oil is produced by steam distillation of the flowering herbs.

Rose
(rosa damascena, r. centifolia, r. gallica)

The deep, sweet, floral bouquet of roses is maybe one of the most profound and symbolic scent of all plants. It is unequivocally associated with feminine beauty and charm. Since ancient times, rose oil has been used as the ultimate aphrodisiac, but it is also relaxing and is a sedative. When applied to the skin, it is a very valuable ingredient for treating inflamed, irritated, dry and sensitive skin. It helps to strengthen and restore broken capillaries and cleans skin impurities. Roses which are suitable for the production of essential oils, are primarily cultivated in France and Eastern Europe. Since the extraction rate is low, rose oils are quite expensive.

Rose Geranium
(pelargonium roseum)

There are numerous different species of odoriferous geraniums. Two of these, the rose and lemon geranium, are the most prominent. Both oils are extracted from the leaves, flowers, and stalks using steam distillation. Rose geranium has a rosy-sweet, minty scent with a cleansing, refreshing, and astringent effect on the skin. In combination with lavender and sandalwood, the bouquet becomes warmer and deeper with a relaxing character. Rose geranium has been reported to have potent antibacterial and antifungal properties, which are useful in formulations for acne, oily skin and greasy hair. It is notable that the Indian or Turkish geranium oil, which has a similar aroma, is not derived from the true geranium (geraniaceae), but from another plant called palmarosa (graminaceae). This oil was described previously.

Rosemary
(rosmarinus officinalis)

Rosemary essential oil is produced by steam distillation of the flowering heads or also from the whole plant. It has a strong, herbaceous, minty-spicy scent with a refreshing, invigorating effect. Rosemary is known to help to relieve headaches. Due to its antimicrobial properties, rosemary oil is effective in the treatment of acne, eczema, dandruff, and greasy hair.

Sandalwood
(santalum album)

The sandalwood tree grows in East India and is well-known for its characteristic strong balm, and sweet odor. This essential oil is extracted from the wood and roots by steam distillation. Sandalwood is widely used in perfumes and skin care products. Its intense scent has a stimulating, invigorating, and also an aphrodisiac effect. It has been found to help to treat itching as well as skin inflammations.

Sage
(salvia officinalis)

Sage is produced by steam distillation from the leaves of the plant. The oil is extensively used as an essential fragrance in perfumes, soaps, creams, and lotions. Sage oil has effective antiseptic and antioxidant properties. In skin and hair care products, it is primarily used to reduce perspiration and to treat insect bites and dandruff.

Sweet Orange
(citrus sinensis)

Dependent upon the selected parts of the fruit, both steam distillation and cold extraction are utilized to produce a sweet orange essential oil. The peel of the fruit is useful as well as the leaves, twigs, and freshly picked flowers. Orange essential oil smells sweet and fruity and has a refreshing effect, particularly in combination with other citric oils. The oil has been known to exhibit antifungal and antibacterial properties. Because of the risk of hyperpigmentations, orange oil should not be applied to sun-exposed skin.

Tea Tree
(melaleuca alternifolia)

Tea tree essential oil is obtained by steam distillation from the leaves and twigs of a small shrub, which is native to Australia. The oil has potent antiseptic properties, and is thus very valuable for the treatment of acne, oily skin, and dandruff. It is also effective in the healing of wounds and helps to cure many different skin diseases.

Thyme
(thymus vulgaris)

This essential oil is extracted by steam distillation from the leaves and flowering tops of the plant, which is originally from the Mediterranean region. The red thyme oil is the crude distillate, while the white thyme oil results from further distillation processes. Thyme oil has a fresh, spicy-herbaceous scent, which is widely used as a fragrance in soaps, creams, and after-shave lotions. It has antiseptic properties and is well-known as a folklore remedy for treating colds and coughs.

Vetiver
(vetiveria zizanioides)

The dark brown essential oil of vetiver is obtained by steam distillation from the tall scented grass and rootlets. The plant is particularly very common in India and Sri Lanka. The deep, smokey, earthy odor of vetiver oil has a relaxing, sedative effect. It is an ideal ingredient in bath oil preparations to produce a relaxing bouquet. In skin care products, vetiver is helpful for acne and oily skin.

Yarrow
(achillea millefolium)

Yarrow, with its white flowers, is commonly found in flowering meadows. This essential oil is produced by steam distillation from the dried herb. It has a fresh herbaceous odor. Yarrow oil has a soothing effect and has good antiinflammatory and antiseptic properties due to its content of azulene. It is used for wounds, sores, acne, and skin rashes. Yarrow, has been suggested as promoting hair growth.

Ylang Ylang
(cananga odorata)

Ylang ylang essential oil is produced by steam distillation from freshly picked flowers. Dependent upon the number of distillations, there are four different grades of oils. The oil derived from the very first distillation is called "extra" and has the highest grade. Further distillates are called grades 1, 2, and 3. Ylang ylang oil is also available as a concrete and an absolute. The scent is exotic, sweet, and floral, and is often used in perfumes as a top note. It has a stimulating and also an aphrodisiac effect. Ylang ylang is very effective in the treatment of oily skin and greasy hair, and has been suggested as promoting hair growth. Caution: at high concentrations, ylang ylang can cause headaches.

Preservatives

Preservatives are added to cosmetic products to inhibit the growth of microorganisms such as bacteria and fungi. Because of the content of water and organic materials, microorganisms can grow rapidly in the absence of antibiotic agents. When bacteria occur at a certain concentration, cosmetic products will spoil and also induce infections, particularly in the eyes and ears. Spoiling is recognized by discoloration, separation of emulsions, and the formation of gas and odors. Thus, preservation is absolutely necessary. Ideally, a preservative is non-irritant, long-lasting, and effective against a wide range of microorganisms.

Many botanical ingredients, such as aloe vera, vitamin C and E, and most essential oils, have good antibacterial, antiviral, and antifungal properties. When used at sufficient concentrations, these natural substances are capable of avoiding spoiling for a few weeks, dependent on the content and type of the product. However, if a shelf life of months or years is desired, as in commercial products, the properties of these natural substances are not effective enough to completely suppress the growth of microorganisms. Therefore, almost all cosmetics on the market are supplemented with synthetic or modified natural preservatives. The following substances are utilized most: formaldehyde and formaldehyde donors (Quaternium-15, Bronopol, DMDM Hydantoin), methylchloro-isothiazolinones (Kathon CG, Euxyl K100), triclosan (Irgasan DP - 300), sorbic acid, benzyl alcohol, and parabens.

In my recipes, I use a product (Germaben-II) which combines two different preservatives, such as parabens and diazolidinyl urea (DiU). These substances are mild and effective against a wide range of microorganisms. Parabens are chemically modified to propyl- and methylparaben, to improve their antibiotic properties. Both propyl- and methylparaben are well-known to be very mild and only rarely cause skin problems. Parabens are less active against bacteria than against yeast and molds. Therefore, diazolidinyl urea is added to assure effective antibacterial activity. Diazolidinyl urea is a formaldehyde derivative and is reported to be non-toxic and non-irritating.

Generally, I use preservatives only in creams and lotions, or in products containing lecithin and/or proteins. While creams and lotions are readily contaminated by the fingers, lecithin and proteins promote bacterial growth. In the recipes in this book, the final concentration of the preservatives is 0.3%. Most commercial products contain a mixture of several different preservatives to achieve a shelf life of two to four years. Such highly concentrated blends have often been found to be responsible for skin irritations and contact dermatitis.

Hence, creating your own cosmetics allows you to shorten the shelf life and to omit or limit synthetic preservatives. In all my recipes containing preservatives, the concentration is calculated for a shelf life of about two months. To obtain a shelf life of about six months, you may use twice the concentration than that indicated. However, I would expect your shampoo or shower gel to be used up before then!

Appendix

References

Cosmetics and Toiletries:
Development, Production, and Use
Wilfried Umbach
1991. Halsted Press, Div. of John
Wiley & Sons, Inc., New York, NY

Principles of Cosmetics for the
Dermatologist
Phillip Frost, Steven N. Horwitz
1982. The C. V. Mosby Company,
St. Louis, MO

Cosmetics, Toiletries, and Health
Care Products
Recent Developments
Georg W. Owens
1978. Noyes Data Corp.,
Park Ridge, NJ

Fisher's Contact Dermatitis
Robert L. Rietschel, Joseph F. Fowler
1995. Williams and Wilkins,
Baltimore, ML

Textbook of Contact Dermatitis
Peter J. Frosch, Richard J. G. Rycroft
1994. Springer Verlag,
New York, NY

Hair and Scalp Disorders
Rodney Dawber, Dominique Van
Neste
1995. J. B. Lippincott Company,
Philadelphia, PA

Unwanted Effects of Cosmetics and
Drugs Used in Dermatology
Johan P. Nater, Anton C. de Groot
1993. Elsevier Science Publishers,
Amsterdam, The Netherlands

Natural Product Medicine.
A Scientific Guide to Foods, Drugs,
and Cosmetics
Ara H. Der Marderosian, Lawrence
E. Liberti
1988. G. F. Stickley Corp.,
Philadelphia, PA

Encyclopedia of Common Natural
Ingredients Used in Food, Drugs,
and Cosmetics
Albert Y. Leung, Steven Foster
1996. Wiley & Sons, Inc.,
New York, NY

The Complete Medicinal Herbal
Penelope Ody
1993. Dorling Kindersley, Inc.,
New York, NY

The Natural Pharmacy
Miriam Polunin, Christopher
Robbins
1992. Maxwell Macmillan
Publishing Company, New York, NY

Your Guide to Standardized Herbal
Products
Rebecca Flynn, Mark Roest
1995. One World Press, Prescott, AZ

Illustrated Encyclopedia of
Essential Oils. The Complete Guide
to the Use of Oils in Aromatherapy
and Herbalism
Julia Lawless
1995. Element Books, Inc.,
Rockport, MA

The Complete Book of Essential
Oils and Aromatherapy
Valerie A. Worwood
1991. New World Library,
Novato, CA

Chemistry and Technology of the
Cosmetics and Toiletries Industry
D. F. Williams
1996. Blackie Academic,
Glasgow, Scotland, UK

Environmental and Human Safety
of Major Surfactants
Sylvia S. Talmage
1994. Lewis Publishers,
Boca Raton, FL

Pharmaceutical Skin Penetration
Enhancement
Kenneth A. Walters and Jonathan
Hadgraft
1993. Marcel Dekker, New York, NY

Cationic Surfactants
James M. Richmond
1990. Marcel Dekker, New York, NY

Biosurfactants and Biotechnology
Naim Kosaric, W. L. Cairns,
Neil C. C. Gray
1987. Marcel Dekker, New York, NY

Surfactants in Cosmetics
Martin M. Rieger
1985. Marcel Dekker, New York, NY

Supplier List

Basic Ingredients

Distilled Water: Local Drug Stores
Sheabutter: Somerset Company;
    Liberty; Henkel; Protameen;
    Terry Laboratories
Xanthan Gum: Somerset Company;
    Henkel; TIC Gum; Liberty

Plant Distillates

Aloe Vera: Local Health Stores;
    Liberty; Terry Laboratories;
    Protameen; CRH International
    Inc.; Mountain Rose Herbs
Orange Flower Water: Local
    Health Stores; Liberty, Aroma
    Vera; Mountain Rose Herbs
Rose Water: Local Health Stores;
    Aroma Vera; Liberty; Mountain
    Rose Herbs
Witch Hazel Water: Local Health
    and Drug Stores; Somerset
    Company; Mountain Rose
    Herbs; American Distilling
    & MFG Inc.

Botanicals and Extracts

Fresh extracts or powdered plants
useful for tinctures are available at
the following companies:

Local Health Stores; Gaia Botanicals;
Gaia Herbs; Green Terrestrial; Herb
Pharm; Moonrise Herbs; Mountain
Rose Herbs; San Francisco Herb Co;
Frontier Herbs; Herb Products Co.

Plant Oils

Almond Oil: Local Health Stores;
    Liberty; Frontier Herbs; LIPO;
    Aroma Vera; Montain Rose
    Herbs; Herb Products Co.
Apricot Kernel Oil: Local Health
    Stores; LIPO; Liberty; Mountain
    Rose Herbs; Herb Products Co.
Avocado Oil: Local Health Stores;
    Liberty; Frontier Herbs; LIPO;
    Henkel; Herb Products Co.
Calendula Oil: Local Health
    Stores; Somerset Company;
    Mountain Rose Herbs; Henkel
Jojoba Oil: Local Health Stores;
    Liberty; Mountain Rose Herbs;
    Protameen; LIPO; R.I.T.A;
    Frontier Herbs; Aroma Vera
Soybean Oil: Local Health Stores,
    Liberty; LIPO
Sunflower Oil: Local Health Stores;
    Liberty; LIPO; Protameen
Wheat Germ Oil: Local Health
    Stores; Liberty; LIPO; R.I.T.A;
    Frontier Herbs; Henkel; Herb
    Products Co.

Vitamins

Vitamin A: Local Health Stores;
   Somerset Company; Henkel
Vitamin C: Local Health Stores;
   Somerset Company
Vitamin E: Somerset Company;
   Henkel; Protameen; Mountain
   Rose Herbs; Local Health Stores
Vitamin B5: Somerset Company;
   R.I.T.A; Protameen

Proteins

Hydrolyzed Soy Protein: Somerset
   Company; Brooks; R.I.T.A

Other Botanical Ingredients

Honey: Local Food Store
Lecithin: Somerset Company;
   R.I.T.A; Liberty

Surfactants

Cocoamidopropyl Betaine: Witco;
   Somerset Company; Henkel;
   Protameen; R.I.T.A;
Potassium Coco Hydrolyzed
   Collagen: Somerset Company;
   Henkel; Brooks; R.I.T.A
Decyl Polyglucose: Somerset
   Company; Henkel
Lauryl Dimonium Hydrolyzed
   Collagen: Somerset Company;
   Henkel; Brooks

Emulsifiers

Polysorbate 80: Lipo; Somerset
   Company; Henkel, Protameen;
   R.I.T.A; Heterene; Witco
Polysorbate 60: Somerset
   Company; Protameen; Lipo;
   Heterene; R.I.T.A.
Sorbitan Stearate: Somerset
   Company; Protameen; Lipo;
   Heterene

Essential Oils

All essential oils used in the recipes
can be purchased at the following
companies: Local Health Stores; Liberty; Frontier; Aroma Vera

Preservatives

Germaben-II: Somerset Company;
   Sutton Laboratories

Cosmetic Containers

First, check your local drug stores.
The following companies are special-
ized in cosmetic containers and offer a broad selection: Alameda; Caliber Packaging Inc.; Olshen's Bottle
Supply; Continental; McKernan

Disinfectants

Rubbing Alcohol: Local Drug
   Stores

Addresses

Alameda Commons Packaging
4445 Enterprise Street
Fremont, CA 94538
Phone: (510) 651 - 0277
Fax: (510) 651 - 2396

American Distilling, MFG Inc.
P. O. Box 319
31 E High Street
East Hampton, CT 06424
Phone: (203) 267 - 4444
Fax: (203) 267 - 1111

Aroma Vera
5901 Rodeo Road
Los Angeles, CA 90016
Phone: (800) 669 - 9514
Fax: (310) 280 - 0395

Brooks Industries, Inc.
70 Tyler Place
South Plainfield, NJ 07080
Phone: (908) 561 - 5200
Fax: (908) 561 - 9174

Caliber Packaging, Inc.
13950 Cerritos Corporate Dr.
Cerritos, CA 90703
Ask for location nearest you
Phone: (800) 737 - 5444
Fax: (310) 802 - 1030

Continental Glass and
Plastic, Inc.
841 West Cermark Road
Chicago, IL 60608 - 4582
Phone: (312) 666 - 2050
Fax: (312) 243 - 3419

CRH International, Inc.
1510 N Parkwood Drive
Harlingen, TX 78550
Phone: (210) 425 - 2926
Fax: (210) 425 - 6264

Frontier Cooperative Herbs
3021 78th Street
P. O. Box 299
Norway, IA 52318
Phone: (800) 786 - 1388
Fax: (319) 227 - 7966

Gaia Botanicals
P. O. Box 8485-A
Philadelphia, PA 19101

Gaia Herbs, Inc.
12 Lancaster County Road
Harvard, MA 01451
Phone: (800) 831 - 7780
         (508) 772 - 5400
Fax: (508) 772 - 5764

Green Terrestrial
P. O. Box 266
Milton, NY 12547
Phone: (914) 795 - 5238

Henkel Corporation
1301 Jefferson Street
Hoboken, NJ 07030
Ask for location nearest you
Phone: (800) 955 - 1456
Fax: (201) 659 - 6698

Herb Pharm
P. O. Box 116
Williams, OR 97544
Phone: (800) 348 - 4372
         (541) 846 - 6262
Fax: (541) 846 - 6112

Herb Products Co.,
P. O. Box 898
North Hollywood, CA 91601
Phone: (818) 984 - 3141

Heterene, Inc.
P. O. Box 247
792 21st Avenue
Paterson, NJ 07543
Phone: (201) 278 - 2000
Fax: (201) 278 - 7512

Liberty Natural Products
8120 SE Stark
Portland, OR 97215
Phone: (800) 289 - 8427
Fax: (503) 256 - 1182

McKernan
Packaging Clearing House
P. O. Box 7281
Reno, NV 89510
Phone: (702) 356 - 6111
Fax: (702) 356 - 2181

Moonrise Herbs
826 G Street
Arcata, CA 95521
Phone: (800) 603 - 8364
Fax: (707) 822 - 0506

Olshen's Bottle Supply
P. O. Box 14627
1204 SE Water Avenue
Portland, OR 97214
Phone: (800) 258 - 4292
Fax: (503) 234 - 8334

Protameen Chemicals, Inc.
375 Minnisink Road
Totowa, NJ 07511
Phone: (201) 256 - 4374
Fax: (201) 256 - 6764

R.I.T.A Corporation (Midwest)
1725 Kilkenny Court
P. O. Box 1487
Woodstock, IL 60098
Phone: (815) 337 - 2500
Fax: (815) 337 - 2522

R.I.T.A Corporation (Northeast)
81 Orchard St.
Ramsey, NJ 07446
Phone: (201) 934 - 0616
Fax: (201) 934 - 0674

R.I.T.A Corporation (Southwest)
4808 Lakawana
Dallas, TX 75247
Phone: (214) 732 - 8964
Fax: (214) 732 - 8964

San Francisco Herb Co.
250 14th Street
San Francisco, CA 94103
Phone: (800) 227 - 4530
Fax: (415) 861 - 4440

Somerset Company
P. O. Box 213
Bellevue, WA 98009
Phone: (425) 649 - 1979
Fax: (425) 649 - 1979

Sutton Laboratories
116 Summit Avenue
P. O. Box 837
Chatham, NJ 07928
Phone: (800) 622 - 4423
Fax: (201) 635 - 4964

Terry Laboratories, Inc.
390 North Wickham Road,
Suite F
Melbourne, Florida 32935
Phone: (800) 367 - 2563
            (407) 259 - 1630
Fax: (407) 242 - 0625

TIC Gums
4609 Richlynn Drive
Belcamp, MD 21017
Phone: (800) 221 - 3953
            (410) 273 - 7300
Fax: (410) 273 - 6469

Witco Corporation
1 American Lane
Greenwich, CT 06831
Phone: (800) 779 - 4826
            (Northeast/West)
            (800) 494 - 8287
            (Southeast/Central)
Fax: (203) 552 - 2850

Index

A

Absolute **75**, 77, 78, 79, 84
Acidity **17**, 25, 46, 55, 70
Ache, muscular 77, 79
Achillea millefolium 83
Acne 60, 62, 63, 64, 65, 76,
    77, 78, 79, 80, 81, 82, 83
After-shave 64, 83
After-sun lotion 39
    recipes 40
Alcohol
    benzyl 85
    ethyl 59
    grain 59
    isopropyl 15
    rubbing 15
Alkalinity **17**, 25, 55, **70**
Allantoin 57, 61
Allergy 17, 66, 70, 71
Almond oil 64
Aloe barbadensis 60
Aloe vera 60
Aloe vulgaris 60
Alpha-bisabolol 76
Althea 63
Ammonium, quaternary
    51, 73
Anionic 51
Antiacneic 58, 60, 62, 63, 65,
    76, 77, 78, 79, 80, 81, 82, 83
Antiaging 62, 66, 67, 68
Antibacterial 19, 22, 50,
    60, 65, 68, 81, 82, 84, 85
Antibiotic 84
Anti-dandruff 47 - 48, 60,
    63, 64, 77 - 82
Antifungal 19, 60, 81, 82, 84
Antiitching 60, 63, 64, 80, 81

Antimicrobial 81
Antioxidant 40, 57, 60, 66, 67,
    68, 82
Antiinflammatory 57, 60, 61,
    62, 63, 64, 67, 68, 76, 77,
    80, 83
Antiseptic 57, 60, 63, 82, 83
Antiviral 19, 84
Anti-wrinkle 62, 66
Aphrodisiac 77, 80, 81, 84
Apigenin 61
Apricot kernel oil 65
Arctium lappa 60
Aromatherapy 75
Ascorbic acid 68
Astringent 57, 60, 63, 64, 76
    80, 81
Avocado oil 65
Azulene 76, 83

B

Bacteria 13, 19, 56, 84, 85
Bacterial growth 50, 85
Bar soap 25, 37
Bath oils 21 - 22
    recipes 23 - 24
    floating 22
    dispersible 22
Benzalkonium chloride 71
Bergamot 76
Betula pendula 60
Biodegradable 72, 73
Birch 60
Bleaching 41, 52
Blow drying 43, 44
Bristles 43
Brushing 41, 43
Burdock 60
Burns 60, 61, 62, 63

C

Cajeput 76
Calendula
    officinalis 62, 65
    oil 65
    tincture 62
Cananga odorata 84
Capillaries 58, 80
Cationic **51**, 73
Centella asiatica 62
Chamaemelum nobile 61
Chamomile
    essential oil 76
    German 61, **76**
    Roman 61, 76
    tincture 61
Chamomilla
    matricaria 61
    recutica 61
Cinnamic ester 57
Citrus aurantium 79
Citrus bergamia 76
Citrus limon 78
Citrus paradisi 77
Citrus sinensis 82
Clary sage 76
Coal tar 48
Cocamido DEA 71
Coco betaine 72
Coco collagen 72
Cocoamidopropyl betaine 72
Co-emulsifier 74
Cold 24, 77, 79, 80, 83
Collagen 53, 68, 69
Collagen, hydrolyzed 73
Collagen quat 52, 73
Coloring 41, 43, 61
Comfrey 61
Concrete 75, 77, 78, 79, 84

Conditioner 46, 51 - 52
    film-forming 51, 52
    recipes 53 - 54
Coneflower, purple 61
Congestion, nasal 24
Contamination 13, 20, 85
Corn oil 66
Cortex 41, 42
Cough 24, 79, 80, 83
Cream 40
Cuticle **41**, 52, 53, 73
Cymbopogon martinii 79

D

Dandruff 47 - 48
    dry 49
    oily 50
    recipes 49 - 50
Decoction, plant 15, **56**
Decyl polyglucose 72
Dermatitis 76
    berloque 76
    contact 19, 60, 85
Diaper 65
Diazolidinyl urea 19, 20, **85**
Disinfection 15
Disodium laureth sulfate 71
Distilled water 15, 17, **55**
Distillate, plant 57
Distillation 17, **55**, 75
DiU, Diazolidinyl urea 19, 20, **85**
Drugs, cytostatic 48

E

Echinacea 61
Echinacea angustifolia 61
Eczema 47, 60, 65, 76, 78, 81
Elastin 69
Electricity, static 41, 51, 53
Emulsion 18
Emulsifier 18, **73**
Equipment 13 - 14
Essential oils 19, 75 - 84
Ester, cinnamic 77

Eucalyptus 77
Eucalyptus globulus 77
Exhaustion, nervous 77
Extract, plant 58
Extract, fluid 58
Eye-irritating 45, 72

F

Face cleansing lotion 35
    recipes 36 - 38
Fatty acids, unsaturated 65, 66
Formaldehyde 85
Fresh water 43
Fungi 84

G

Germaben-II 20, 85
Gin, dry 59
Ginseng 62
Glands, sebaceous 38, 45
Gotu kola 62
Grapefruit 77

H

Hair 41 - 343
    blond 61
    breakage 43
    brush 43
    conditioner 51 - 52
    damaged 42, 51, 52, 53
    dry 44
    dye 42, 43
    fullness 51, 53
    graying 63
    greasy 45, 76, 81, 84
    growth 62, 77, 83, 84
    loss 60, 64, 78
    rinse 54
    shine 41, 51, 52, 53, 73
    structure 41
    unproblematic 46
Hair shampoo 41 - 43
    recipes 44 - 46

Hamamelis virginiana 64
Hand cleanser 25 - 26
    recipes 27 - 28
Hand mixer 15
Headache 24, 45, 77, 80, 81, 84
Healing 57, 60, 62, 63, 64 65,
    68, 79, 82
Helpful tips 15 - 20
Honey 69
Humectant 69, 71
Hydrolipid 17, 37
Hydrolysate 69
Hydrophilic 70, 73
Hypericum perforatum 64
Hyperkeratosis 67
Hyperpigmentation 76, 78, 82

I

Infant 45
Infection 19, 77, 78, 79, 84
Inflammation 11, 17, 47, 50, 60,
    62, 65, 70, 79, 80, 81
Infusion, plant 56
Ingredients 55 - 85
    basic 17, 55 - 57
Itching 60, 63, 64, 80, 81

J

Jasmine 77
Jasminum grandiflorum 77
Jojoba oil 65
Juniper berry 78
Juniper communis 78

K

Keratin 52, 69
Keratinization 67
Kernel oil 64, 65

L

Lauramido DEA 71
Lauryl dimonium -
    hydrolyzed collagen 73

Lavender 78
Lavendula officinalis 78
Lecithin 20, **70**, 85
Lemon 78
Lemon balm 78
Lemon juice 17, **70**
Lipophilic 70, 73

M
Maleleuca alternifolia 82
Maleleuca leucadendron 76
Mantle
    acid 17, 25, 37, 55, 70
    fatty 71
Marigold
    oil 65
    tincture 62
Marsh mallow 63
Matricaria chamomilla 76
Matricaria recutica 76
Melanin 42
Melissa officinalis 78
Mentha piperita 80
Methylchloroisothiazo-
    linone 85
Microcirculation 64
Microorganisms 19, 84
Mineral oil 21, 66
Mineral salts 55
Mixer 15
Moisturizing 57, 60, 63, 67,
    68, 69, 70
Monosaccharide 69

N
Nausea 80
Nourishing 21, 40, 65, 66

O
Olive oil 66
Orange flower water 57
Origanum marjorana 79

P
Palmarosa 79
Panax ginseng 62
Panthenol 68
Paraben 19, 20, **85**
    methyl 85
    propyl 85
Patchouli 80
Pelargonium roseum 81
Perspiration 63, 82
pH-value 70
Phospholipid 42, 70
Plant
    decoction 56
    distillate 57
    extract 58
    infusion 56
Plantago major 63
Plantain 63
Pogostemon cablin 80
Polyglucose 72
Polymer, synthetic 52
Polyoxyethlene 74
Polysaccharide 69
Polysorbate (60) 18, **74**
Polysorbate (80) 18, **74**
Preservative 19, 20, 84 - 85
Procedure 15 - 16
Proliferation, cell 62
Protein 69
    hydrolyzed 52, 69, 72
Psoriasis 61
Purple coneflower 61

Q
Quat 51, 73

R
Radiation, solar/UV 25, 39,
    43, 57, 65, 67, 68
Radicals, free 66, 67, 68
Radix althaea 63

Rash 62, 65, 76, 83
Regenerating 35, 61, 62,
    65, 70
Relaxing 23, 32, 77, 78, 79,
    80, 81, 83
Retinol 67
Rinse 54
Rosa centifolia 80
Rosa damascena 80
Rosa gallica 80
Rose 80
Rose geranium 81
Rose water 58
Rosemarinus officinalis 81
Rosemary 81
Rubbing alcohol 15

S
Safflower oil 66
Sage
    essential oil 82
    tincture 63
Salicylic acid 48
Salt water 34, 43
Salvia officinalis 63, 82
Salvia sclarea 76
Sandalwood 81
Santalum album 81
Scales 41, 47, 48, 50
Scalp 42, 43, 47
    dry 47
    oily 47, 78
Sebaceous glands 38, 45
Seborrhea 45, 78, 79
Sebum 44, 50, 51
Selenium sulfide 48
Sesame oil 66
Sheabutter 18, **57**
Shelf life 19, 85
Shower gel 29 - 30
    recipes 31 - 34
Side-effects 11, 42

Skin
    acneic 60, 62, 63, 64,
        65, 76, 77, 78, 79,
        80, 81, 82, 83
    aging 57, 58, 69
    baby 24
    chapped 28, 39
    dry 28, 32, 37, 58, 61, 77,
        78, 80
    infection 19, 77, 78, 79, 84
    inflammation 11, 17, 47,
        60, 62, 65, 79, 81
    irritation 17, 19, 25, 43,
        60, 62, 63, 68, 70,
        71, 72, 79, 80, 85
    oily 77, 81, 82, 83, 84
    rash 62, 65, 76, 83
    sensitive 28, 32, 37, 58,
        61, 77, 78, 80
    ulcer 61, 62
Soap
    bar 25, 37
    liquid 11, **25**, 26, 71
Sodium 17, 25, 55
Sodium lauryl sulfate 71
Sodium laureth sulfate 71
Soothing 34, 39, 40, 57, 58,
    60, 61, 63, 64, 65, 76,
    77, 79, 83
Sorbic acid 85
Sorbitan ester 74
Sorbitan stearate 18, **74**
Sore 24, 76, 77, 79
Soy protein 69
Soybean oil 66
Sperm whale oil 65, 66
Spermaceti oil 65
Split ends 41, 52
Spoiling 19, 60, 65, 67, 68, 84
St. John's wort 64
Sting 63
Stinging Nettle 64
Stress 77

Sunburn 39, 58, 60, 63, 64, 78
Sun exposure 39, 40, 43, 76,
    78, 82
Sunflower oil 66
Surfactants 18, 71 - 73
    amphoteric 72
    cationic 51, 73
    film-forming 51
    non-ionic 72
    protein-conjugated 51
Sweet orange 82
Symphytum officinale 61
Syndet 71

T

Tanning 39
Tea 17, **56**
Tea tree 82
Thickener 15, **56**, 69, 74
Thyme 83
Thymus vulgaris 83
Tincture 58
Tips 17 - 20
Tocopherol 67
Toner 35
    recipes 36 - 38
Triclosan 85

U

Unsaponifiable 57
Urtiga dioica 64
Utensils, cooking 13 - 14

V

Vetiver 83
Vetiveria zizanioides 83
Viscosifier 71
Vitamin A 67
Vitamin B5 68
Vitamin C 68
Vitamin E 67
Vitamin, fat-soluble 67

Vitamin, water-soluble 68
Vodka 59

W

Wash activity 18
Water
    demineralized 55
    distilled 15, 17, **55**
    fresh 43
    orange flower 57
    rose 58
    salt 34, 43
    tap 17, 55, 56
    temperature 43, 56, 71
    witch hazel 58
Waving 41, 52
Wax 65, 74, 75
Weathering 44, 51, 52
Wheat germ oil 66
Witch hazel
    tincture 63
    water 58
Wound 57, 60, 61, 62, 63,
    68, 79, 82

X

Xanthan gum 15, **56**
Xanthomonas campestris 56

Y

Yarrow 83
Ylang ylang 84

Z

Zinc pyrithione 48

About the Author

Karin Bombeli grew up in Zurich, Switzerland. For several years, she worked as a nurse in many different hospitals. She always took a keen interest in herbalism and cosmetics. Motivated by her clinical experience with the high incidence of adverse skin reactions due to commercial cosmetics, she continuously extended her knowledge about the dermatological effects of cosmetics. This culminated in the desire to produce her own cosmetics exclusively based on mild and natural ingredients. After having graduated in several college courses regarding the production and technology of cosmetics and toiletries, her hobby finally became her profession. For the last seven years, she has developed her own cosmetic line, which has met with an enthusiastic response. During this time, Karin moved to the USA, where she has started her own business with natural cosmetics. Karin is member of the American Herb Association.

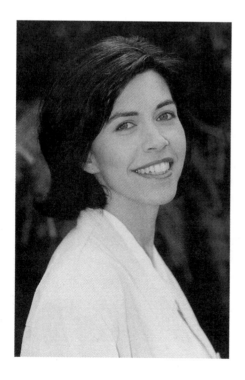